THE
AZTEC WAY
TO
HEALTHY
EATING

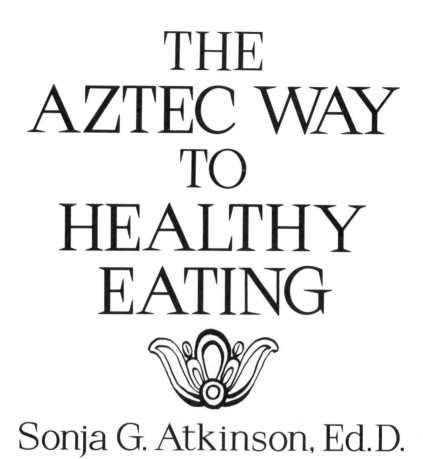

THE
AZTEC WAY
TO
HEALTHY
EATING

Sonja G. Atkinson, Ed.D.

PARAGON HOUSE
New York

First edition, 1992

Published in the United States by

Paragon House
90 Fifth Avenue
New York, N.Y. 10011

Book design by Deirdre C. Amthor

Library of Congress Cataloging-in-Publication Data

Atkinson, Sonja G.,
The Aztec way to healthy eating/by Sonja G. Atkinson.
—1st ed.
p.   cm.
Includes index.
ISBN 1-55778-414-0
1. Aztecs—Food. 2. Aztecs—Nutrition. 3. Aztecs—
Social life and customs. 4. Diet—Mexico. 5. Nutrition
—Mexico.   I. Title.
F1219.3.F64A85   1992
394.1'2'0972—dc20   91-19334
                                                                    CIP

This book is dedicated to my husband,
Gaynor, and my children, Sarah, Daniel,
and Melody, who gave me love and support
through the years of research and effort
involved in the project.

Acknowledgment

I wish to acknowledge my agent, Janet Dight, who has been my mentor and guide, shepherding this work from its hopeful but frail beginning to its conclusion, giving unstintingly of her time and sharing her considerable writing expertise.

Contents

Introduction

My father, an agronomist, spent much of his career working for the United Nations, and our family lived and traveled extensively in Central and South America. I therefore attended bilingual schools, in which students were taught to write papers or discuss any subject in both Spanish and English. In college I majored in Latin American Studies, which provided opportunities to use my bilingual training to further study the people of the lands where I had grown up.

My father was intensely dedicated to educating and helping the farmers in those countries to increase their food production. Farming, soil-improvement techniques, and food quality were the subjects of many conversations in our home.

These two areas of my life did not converge until I was settled with a family that included a youngster who was very sensitive to different chemical substances in foods. My husband and I found ourselves studying all sorts of manuals and reports on nutrition and how it relates to good health. The more I learned from this research, the more it triggered recollections of what I had studied and learned about the way of life of the early Latin American civilizations.

I discovered clues that led to my interpretation of the foods of the Aztec Way in the library at the University of New Mexico. It was always quiet there, permeated with that wonderful musty smell of shelf upon shelf of books. The wide, golden-oak tables glowed under the green-shaded reading lights. I envied the people seated so comfortably at those tables, reading clearly printed books in English.

I would pick up my bulky canisters of microfilm and slowly climb the stairs to the second floor, where the microfilm readers were. The most reliable was Number 2. Its light gray looked unassuming, but it hulked over the small desk, never leaving quite enough room for all my papers. I pressed the ON switch and the familiar whir of the fan helped me focus my expectations. I threaded the film and cranked it to where I had left off. The old Spanish words in tall, spidery handwriting with ostentatious flourishes were difficult to read at first. Then my eyes and my thoughts would concentrate on the task, and I could make sense of the words, then sentences. Soon pictures formed in my mind of the Aztec people and the riches and glories of their empire.

The lively images that formed so readily came from stories, notes, and studies made by the early Spanish explorers. But these men were not the exact object of my study. My actual assignment was to help my Meso-american history professor, Dr. Franz Scholes, research the tactics of Spanish army commanders: I was to find references to the army's muni-tions movements in its effort to control a geographically difficult expanse of territory. I didn't even write down the microfilm number and catalog page for the little personal reference made in a diary by a hungry, dis-gruntled soldier to the effect that "Today is the heathen [Aztec] day they call Monkey, so there is nothing to eat but fruit."

I emerged from the library into an exhilaratingly beautiful New Mex-ico autumn afternoon. The intense turquoise of the Southwestern sky made a vivid backdrop to the soft adobe color of the building—a scene of sky and earth that had not changed since the times I had just been reading about. I began walking under the golden cottonwoods that lined the long path to the parking lot. My thoughts turned to the practical needs of the day, but that tiny fragment of information stayed in my mind. I kept coming back to it, feeling that it would prove the key to something interesting and delightful.

It was several years before other, similar bits of information began to form a pattern and answer questions I'd begun to have about Aztec health, longevity, and life-style. George C. Valiant's book *The Aztecs* gave very clear accounts of the control religion had of Aztec life. Bernal Diaz del Castillo, a soldier who accompanied Cortés in 1520, offered a firsthand report of Aztec life in *The Bernal Diaz Chronicles*, also empha-sizing the religious fervor that characterized the Aztec people. I read detailed descriptions of Aztec foods and food-preparation methods in the scholarly reports of Fray Bernardino de Sahagun in his *General History of the Things of New Spain.*

The clue I had gotten from the soldier's diary about Day Monkey was just that—a clue. Nowhere in the materials I studied did I find a guide that spelled out in detail what food each day of the Aztec calendar demanded. I do believe that the Aztecs governed their foods by their calendar; that fits with all the information I have about Aztec life in general and about their use of food. I did not find documentation for every individual day of their twenty-day calendar, but once I had the concept in mind, I was able to fill in the gaps, and a pattern emerged. It was a healthy pattern, a wise pattern based on the ancient wisdom of a great culture.

The materials I read made it clear that the Aztecs developed a highly successful life-style that used the foods of their world to tremendous advantage. And their use of foods formed parallels with what I knew about today's health issues and nutrition research. Articles and books on the effects of fiber, cholesterol, low fat, and fresh fruits and vegetables in our diet have appeared in greater numbers, and the more I studied the Aztec foodstyle, the more I realized that the positive principles they discovered have not changed with time. The natural products of the earth, used in a defined system, succeed as well today as they did seven hundred years ago.

It was difficult for me to remain objective about the information I was able to gather and organize. I was amazed, and I developed a delighted enthusiasm for what I was finding. I found that the Aztec system is the world's first rotation diet, because of the twenty-day cycle of the Aztec calendar. It uses a healthy combination of some meat dishes and alternate protein sources. The twenty days of the calendar alternate various kinds of foods in a way that makes nutritional sense *and* keeps one's palate entertained.

I began to see the Aztec Way as a panacea for almost all the dietary ills we suffer. We are warned about the high fat content of our contemporary diet. The Aztec foods use few fats and oils. We hear about possible dangers from too many sweets and too much refined sugar. The Aztecs had no refined sugar, and the recipes in this book do not call for it. There is mounting concern about the glut of red meat in our diet. The Aztecs ate few red meats since they did not have cattle. We are encouraged to eat fruits and vegetables. The Aztecs saw these foods as their source of strength, and they are used consistently in the Aztec meals. Finally, there is growing wariness about our high consumption of artificial preservatives and colors and flavors. The Aztec foods are simple and basic and use few preprepared foods.

The Aztec foodstyle is also a wonderful answer for the many people allergic to wheat and milk products. In its basic menus it is a tasty way to have a wheat-free life-style, not just a dish or two that does not have wheat. Because the Aztecs didn't have cattle, most of the menus are also milk- and cheese-free. I had friends who needed just that foodstyle, and their reaction was one of delight as they finally had menus of interesting, positive things to eat instead of an unsettling list of foods to avoid.

This book also provides a means to understand some of the spiritual connection the Aztecs, who were so closely bonded to the natural world around them, had with the nurturing bounty of Mother Earth.

Note to the Reader

This book is divided into three sections: the Aztecs; Aztec foods and nutrition today; menus and recipes.

1. The first three chapters tell a little about Aztec life so that you can see why the correlation between the foods of the Aztecs, their way of life, and their calendar makes sense. The Aztecs were an intensely religious people, and their religion dictated much of what happened in their lives. The Aztec calendar is a powerful symbol of their religion and is the twenty-day rotation that dictated their foods.

2. Chapters 4 and 5 deal with Aztec foods themselves, especially the benefits of the Aztec foodstyle and how it meets our needs today in such an effective way. No matter how interesting or exotic any particular food plan may seem, if it is to have any value, it must be nutritionally sound. We have received good counsel over and over not to attempt extreme fad diets. A close look at the nutritional values of Aztec foods makes clear that this foodstyle is not a flimsy fad but a sound and satisfying way to eat that offers zesty alternatives to more standard health fare.

The valuable, health-giving foods of the Aztecs and the way they were arranged and cooked are very adaptable for our benefit today. Creative use of fresh fruits and vegetables, few fats, and high natural fiber make these foods, and the way they were eaten in a specific order, a great resource in our health-conscious times.

3. Chapter 6, on menus, suggests specific foods for each of the twenty days of the Aztec calendar. The glyph for each day is shown, with a poem that gives the thought or mood of that day's character.

Our kitchen-tested recipes (Chapter 7) use ingredients available in most stores in most parts of the country. Once you are familiar with the menus, you may want to experiment with your own favorite recipes or recipes similar to the ones suggested in the book. But be sure to maintain the healthy cooking style of the Aztecs, which used little fats and frying.

I have a sincere wish for you as you follow the suggestions in this book: *Have fun!* I did, because I became so enthusiastic about this project. It has taken four years to develop, and the help of many people, especially my family (who lived through the disastrous recipes that *didn't* get published) and my teacher and agent, Janet Dight, who made it possible to get these ideas expressed in a readable way. I think the Aztec foodstyle can be applied beneficially to our lives today, especially if you give it time. Any natural, diet-related change in your life is often subtle and slow, not the instant, overnight sensation we wish it would be. The key is the Aztec calendar, which gives the rotation, the variety, and the meaning to this unique foodstyle.

A book that was particularly inspiring to me in this process was *Mexico: A History in Art* by Bradley Smith. It beautifully portrays the Aztecs' powerful works of art, their poetry, their mysticism, and their focus on their religion.

1
An Aztec Feast Day

A quiet group of people stands at the base of one of the small ceremonial pyramids near the center of the capital city of Tenochtitlán (TEN-ohk-tee-tlahn). The flattened top of the pyramid rises a little over one story high, and the voice of the priest is easily heard as he intones the familiar songs:

> The heat of the sun strikes
> Mother Earth
> With the power of fertility
> And the strength of growth;
> I yearn for Life Rain
> To penetrate her sweetness
> As my sweat waters the corn
>
> *Aztec Song for Rain*

> A woman with child kneels and
> Cries in her travail.
> There is wetness now
> Upon the earth, and blood,
> And new life.
>
> *Song of Life*

The songs end as a welcome cloud momentarily covers the midday sun. A drum begins the rhythm of the final chant for the ceremony:

I am connected with all the life around me. Life Rain brings food from Mother Earth. Inside the pale inner leaves of the husk, the golden Sun Seeds of corn nestle in living strands of silver silk.

The power of life surrounds me. Vibrant power lies in the plants and animals that are my meat. I see power in the wind, the water, and the moon.

All things are in a circle. I am in the circle of Mother Earth and the heavens.

The chanting ceases, the last notes seeming to float and fade slowly. The Aztec priest remains in front of the stone altar, arms stretched to the sky, until the resonant drumming ends. The ceremonial fire burns in a sacred hollow of red sandstone next to the altar. The priest now adds copal incense to the coals, making a pungent cloud billow toward the sky to carry the songs and chants to the heavens.

There is little room at the top of the pyramid. The tall priest and the two drummers move solemnly, carefully to end the prayer ritual. The drummers carry the long drum log slowly down the steep steps of the pyramid. They wear ceremonial turquoise loincloths, sandals, and a simple headdress with one long bright-blue feather above each ear.

The priest also descends slowly; the steps are so shallow that he must place his sandaled feet sideways on each one. His woven mantle forms a train of color behind him, contrasting with the vivid purple loincloth that marks his high priestly rank.

Reaching the cobbled street, the priest walks three blocks toward the main pyramid. It is a much larger building, standing more than six stories high. Engineered with great accuracy, the broad base spans eighty feet and is within fractions of an inch to true level. White limestone blocks, hewn with great skill, slope in steep steps to the top platform. Bold carvings of plumed serpents cascade down the sides of the main steps, their symmetry and intricate detail sharply outlined in the returning sunshine.

Other priests have gathered at the corner of the cobbled street, and they greet each other with slight bows. They move their heads slowly and a little stiffly under the weight of their elaborate headdresses. Each headpiece is adorned with rows of beautifully hued and matched feathers, hammered gold to cover the forehead, and carefully carved gold pendants hanging to the shoulders.

They stand, talking quietly, looking at the throngs of people crowding the open square in front of the great pyramid. It is the day of Jaguar on the Aztec calendar, a feast day, a holiday, a day of carnival and celebration.

A shout of approval from the crowd interrupts their conversation, and they climb onto the lower tier of the pyramid for a clearer view. Several acrobats have mounted a platform erected near the center of the square. A small drum and two flutes sound a fast tempo as the acrobats begin a series of jumps, balancing on one another's shoulders and heads. A young girl lies on her stomach across the joined outstretched arms of two young men. Slowly she arches her back, raising her feet until they touch her head and then slide down next to her shoulders. Shouts of approval follow the trilling of the flutes that indicates the end of her act. Three jugglers begin an intricate set of exchanges, and the crowd chants in unison with the drums to encourage the performers.

A commotion starts at the edge of the square as people give way to form a respectful path for a strong, muscular figure striding toward the central pyramid. Slender thongs of jaguar skin hang from a wide belt cinching his deep-blue loincloth. A jaguar pelt hangs down his broad back. He carries a rectangular athlete's pouch containing his sacred collection of feathers and animal entrails that promise to continue his luck in the games.

Four servants follow him in single file, carrying bundles on their heads and shoulders. They are followed by a dejected barefoot figure whose hands are tied before him. His own obvious strength and conditioning form a discordant contrast to his reluctant, shuffling walk and bowed head.

The crowd murmurs as the leader of this small parade passes, and several of the young men reach out respectfully to touch his shoulder, hoping to improve their own fortunes in that lucky touch.

"Ah, the famous Four Jaguar," says one of the priests. "He has a way of exciting the crowd every time he plays."

"Yes," says the tall priest. "And the bettors, too. Just last week four nobles presented their own champion and bet four feather bundles and two jaguar skins on him. They were disgraced when he lost, for they could not cover the bet. They are now slaves to Red Vulture."

"And all that did," comments his friend, "was increase the stakes. Many are sure he cannot possibly win another game. They ask me for omens, and I have nothing clear. Except that it is foolish to wager on sports contests!" His friends laugh in agreement.

"He comes today, the day for which he was named, to make offerings. A pleasant boost to our coffers," says the first priest.

"I wish him continued success," says the tall priest. "And that for his sake, not ours."

Four Jaguar stops directly in front of one of the pyramid's massive carvings of a serpent's head, its mouth open to show exaggerated fangs, stylized feathers forming a ruff around its neck. Crossing his hands over his chest, Four Jaguar begins a short, loud chant. When he finishes, he extends his arms. Quickly the first servant behind him opens his bundle to reveal three sheaves of long, shimmering feathers and carefully places these in Four Jaguar's hands. Four Jaguar then places them atop the stone head before him. A collective sigh of admiration comes from the crowd. Aware of the approving looks of the priests and the interest of the crowd, Four Jaguar again extends his arms, and the second servant gives him a large and beautifully woven cape. Another sigh comes from those around him as he drapes this over the carved feathers. The cloth falls in graceful, exquisitely colored folds. The third and fourth servants now come forward and open their smaller bundles, wrapped carefully in banana leaves. Four molded rounds of precious copal incense are added to the offerings.

Silent anticipation grips the crowd as Four Jaguar motions to his bound opponent, vanquished only yesterday. His face revealing no emotion, the defeated athlete kneels. From his wide belt Four Jaguar draws an obsidian knife. The shiny black stone has been so carefully worked that the keen edge is a translucent gray. Reaching down with his left hand, Four Jaguar grasps the long forelock representing this man's status and freedom. In one swift move, Four Jaguar severs the forelock and part of the scalp beneath. He places this in front of the other offerings, and a bright rivulet of blood trickles down the cream-colored stone. No sound escapes the kneeling figure, now permanently marked a slave to the priests who maintain and clean the pyramids.

The crowd shouts with satisfaction, pleased both with the athlete's gesture and with the stoicism of the victim. The athlete mounts the lower step and faces his admirers. A noble with an orange loincloth and a headdress of orange and yellow feathers joins him and motions to the crowd for silence.

"A poem!" he exclaims. "A poem for Four Jaguar to honor his victory and his fine offering."

A rippling breeze flares the noble's cape. He raises one hand, then pauses before speaking, teasing the silent audience, letting their anticipation build.

> Jaguar with jade-green eyes,
> Crouching in jade-green leaves
> I, too, am ready to leap,
> In power of sun-warmed sinews.
> A growl, a cry,
> Then run, exult in joy of triumph.

Calls of approval come from the crowd. The young noble leaves the step and returns to his cheering friends. Four Jaguar remains for a moment, acknowledging the adulation of the crowd.

"Fortunate omens must have guided the choice of his name," says the tall priest.

"Indeed!" says his friend. "For he displays the graces of the jaguar admirably. Power, grace, and beauty are his. The spirit of the jaguar walks with him."

"A note of envy?" chides the tall one. "Come now! You know his success is due to more than his birth under good omens. I respect the work I know he does to maintain his skills. I also respect how carefully he observes all the rules of the Sun Stone."

Poised in the bright sunlight, skin glistening with palm oil, the athlete represents an Aztec ideal. Of medium stature, he has conditioned his body for feats of skill and endurance. Like his namesake, he is lithe, with quick reflexes and great energy. And he does, as the priest said, carefully follow the rules of the Sun Stone, for he, more than most, wishes for the power of each day, gained when the foods of that day are eaten.

Four Jaguar raises his arms, forms fists, and touches his chest in a salute to the crowd. Then he jumps off the step and swings back through the crowd, his four servants following quickly behind him.

The tall priest watches as his two friends gather the offerings of Four Jaguar. The new slave is still kneeling, his wound still bleeding. One of the priests unties his hands, then gives him several of the smallest banana leaves that had wrapped the incense.

"Here," he says, "cover your head, then come with me."

Three singers and one drummer mount the platform and begin a popular song, but the enthusiasm of the crowd is gone. The tantalizing aromas of the foods of this feast day are drawing people to the food stalls along the wide streets leading to the market square. People begin conversing and moving about, heading down the streets where most of the stalls are set up. Banana leaves hold moist mounds of sweet ground maize flour. The practiced hands of the women quickly and deftly turn these balls of dough into tortillas. These are laid on flat, fire-heated rocks to bake, then placed in a steaming stack to be served. Sweet ears of corn roasted in the husk are opened, and slices of fresh squash dipped in a dark-red chili sauce lie in spicy overlapping circles. One merchant was able to hire runners to bring baskets of mangoes from the lowlands. Even at the high prices he must charge, his stall is soon emptied of the stringy, sweet fruit. Several stands do a brisk business in sweet pockets, rounds of dough filled with honeyed spiced pumpkin. Sounds of laughter and bargaining fill the street.

The main square seems unexpectedly empty as the priests take leave of one another. The tall priest is suddenly aware of the weight of his headdress and the hot twinges of fatigue in the muscles at the base of his neck. He walks quickly along the clean, wide streets, anxious to be resting within the whitened adobe walls of his home. He thinks of his own feast with pleasant anticipation. Because of his high rank he has been able to obtain a talented cook as one of his servants. Today, the day of Jaguar, he will have turkey meat simmered in a sweet but spicy golden sauce and served with tender ears of corn and thin corn cakes. The cook will have prepared a fine vegetable broth and savory beans. He will end his meal with pumpkin and honey nestled inside half-moons of dough.

In spite of these pleasant thoughts, he still feels restless. Turning to his left, he walks again toward the center of this great capital city, seat of the Aztec empire. He reaches a low pyramid, its wide, flattened top only five steps above the ground. At its center rests the great dark-gray rock that is the Sun Stone.

Sixteen of the emperor's honor guard surround the pyramid, four across the bottom of each set of steps that ascend each of the four sides of the pyramid. Recognizing the rank and headdress of the tall priest, two guards stand aside to allow him to climb the pyramid. Reaching the top, he walks to the curved edge of the huge rock. He puts his hand on it and stands in quiet meditation. His eyes do not need to see the brightly painted symbols carved in the stone, for as his hand touches the stone he forms a clear picture of them in his mind. The circle of the sun in the circle of the days in the circle of the symbols of mankind's history. Circles and cycles in an infinite round. He bows in reverence, then descends and turns toward home, his heart at peace, his world in order.

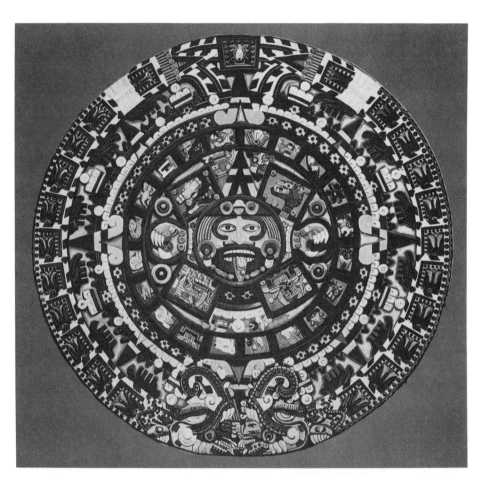

2
The Aztecs

They came from farther north around A.D. 1200, these fierce, loyal, passionate, sensitive Aztecs. Their original home was Aztlan, said to be an island of spiritual power. In reality it was probably a marginally successful agricultural valley whose inhabitants had paid tribute to the Toltecs for many generations. The Aztecs retained their identity in the disintegration of the Toltec empire, which had begun about A.D. 950 and lasted until 1200, and also retained their language, Nahuatl (NAH-wah-ttl).

They were a scraggly band when they first reached the reed-lined shores of Lake Texcoco, which covered part of what is now Mexico City. Their new neighbors, the Texcocos, tolerated them since they did not regard the Aztecs, in their fiber loincloths and fiber sandals, armed with simple bows and stone knives, as much of a threat. The Aztecs' other neighbors, the Tepanecs, were not happy with the newcomers and soon attacked them, almost destroying the tribe. The Tepanecs allowed the survivors to live in a swampy area just north of today's Mexico City, thinking they would likely not survive the snakes infesting the area. Contrary to expectations, the Aztecs flourished by roasting and eating the snakes.

This story typifies the Aztecs' approach to survival. They used everything around them, turning seeming disadvantages into advantages. They borrowed, copied, and adapted anything that would help them survive or would enhance their tribal image.

They settled on the islands of Lake Texcoco, establishing on the largest one their capital city of Tenochtitlán. They began forging their empire in 1325 in a series of violent military conquests.

The Aztecs were surrounded by the Tepanecs, the Texcocos, and the kingdom of Culhuacan (Cool-wah-KAHN), the last of the Toltecs. In a series of skillfully diplomatic moves, the Aztecs constantly made and broke alliances with these tribes to keep them at war with each other so they would not form a defensive alliance against the newcomers. Other, smaller tribes were made vassals and had to pay heavy tribute to their new lords.

A series of highly advanced cultures in this region—the Mayans, Olmecs, and Toltecs—had left a great religious and scientific legacy. True to form, the Aztecs adopted and built on this rich heritage, creating a culture that mixed refinement and barbarity, sensitivity and fanaticism, poetry and passion, prosperity and great governmental strength. They became masters of a land whose loveliness had inspired poets, artists, and mystics for many generations preceding them.

The Aztecs did everything with great intensity and were especially zealous about their religion, which dominated Aztec life. Their religious leaders were their government leaders as well, and from the earliest founding of their empire no major governmental decision was made without seeking the will or guidance of the major Aztec deities. The emperor was considered godlike, having the privilege of communicating directly with the deities of their pantheon or demanding specific answers through a priest. This gave him unquestioned power and total authority.

The concept of sacrifice was central to Aztec religion. The Aztecs believed that at one time in the history of the universe, the earth was in danger of being destroyed. The gods sacrificed themselves so that the universe would not be dissolved. Their power to do good and bring life was in the blood of man also, so the blood of man was the only blood that could return strength to the gods, especially to the sun god Tonatiuh (Toh-NOT-ee-you), who kept the sun in the sky. Drops of blood gathered from nicking one's own earlobe, lip, or finger were the offerings that accompanied sincere prayer. Human sacrifice represented the solemn and sacred culmination of true worship.

In a hundred years the original small band of nomads that came to Lake Texcoco had become powerful rulers. Montezuma I reigned, and his armies had just conquered what today are the states of Puebla, Veracruz, and Morelos. Montezuma's armies were the armed guard of the government and were seen as the armed strength of the gods. His warriors became national heroes. Strength, bravery, cunning, and fierceness were lavishly rewarded, and battlefield promotions in rank became the way many a commoner moved up in status and acquired wealth. The names of the outstanding warriors were sung in poems, their deeds were lauded, their newfound wealth advertised. The very best pressed forward to serve. They were brave, competitive, and fiercely loyal to the emperor who was so loyal to them. Physical strength and endurance became a national aspiration, not just for warriors, but also for those with other careers, especially athletes.

The Aztecs kept careful chronicles of events in their history. How accurately the events are portrayed is questionable, however, since one ruler, Itzcoatl, had the old histories destroyed and new histories written. A reference to this appears in a type of Aztec book, called a *codex*, that uses pictures as writing. The *Codex Matritense* says:

> Their history was preserved.
> But then it was burned.
> When Itzcoatl reigned in Mexico.
> A resolution was taken.
> The lords of the Mexicans said:
> it is not fitting that all people
> should know these pictures.
> Those who are subject, the people,
> will be spoiled
> and the land will be twisted,
> because many lies are preserved in
> those books
> and many in them have been held as gods.

Even if the record of the events is changed, the pictures themselves are a treasure since they reveal so much of Aztec life. The Aztecs are depicted at war, at peace, at worship, at markets, at feasts, at marriage and funeral ceremonies, at home taking care of children.

The Spanish conquerors were also prolific recordkeepers. The conquistador Hernán Cortés sent five letters about the New World back to the king in Spain. But his motives hampered his accuracy as a field reporter: The "facts" he presented to seek approval and additional money were colored by his wish to have the only royal license to explore New Spain. To emphasize his need for increased men, arms, and supplies, for instance, he dwelt at length on the horrifyingly idolatrous nature of the Aztecs, particularly their human sacrifices.

Bartolomé de Las Casas gives a clearer report with quite a different slant. He disagreed with the policy of conquering the Indians first and then converting them. He felt religious conversion should come by peaceful means, and in justifying this view he described many aspects of Aztec life.

Bernadino de Sahagún, an excellent field reporter, wrote a monumental work in which he described Aztec culture in careful detail, including some of their foods, cooking methods, and utensils. These Spanish references have provided much of what we know and much of what is in this book. (Good translations of these works are available, and readers interested in an in-depth look at Aztec life will enjoy them.)

Valuable as these reports are, it is through the Aztecs' own artwork that we can picture them best. As I look at the artwork that survives, especially the sculpture, I visualize clearly the lives of the Aztec people.

They were healthy, fit, and personally very clean. From the way they drew and carved human figures, it is easy to see that they admired athletic skill and strength. Warriors, athletes, dancers, nursing women, and young nobles are well represented in Aztec art. They differ in poses and styles, but they all share a wonderful vitality.

And how they loved adornment! They adorned themselves, their buildings, their pottery, even their daily utensils. And they loved color. They used vivid dyes in the cloth they wove, bright paints in the grand murals on their buildings, and brilliantly colored precious bird feathers on their elaborate headdresses. The Aztecs were a beautiful, mystical people; part of a beautiful, mystical land.

When they needed to chronicle their accomplishments accurately, and to make sure they were honoring their gods properly and in correct order, the Aztecs looked for a calendar. Using their characteristic energy and acquisitiveness, they adapted the Mayan concept of organizing the changing of the seasons (equinoxes, solstices) and the passing of time into a calendar. They used their own dating method and their own gods. The calendar provided a numbering system, a canvas upon which to show the major events in their cosmos, and dictated the cycles of ceremonial worship.

The Aztec Calendar

The Great Sun Stone, the Aztec calendar, inspires awe in all who stand before it. It measures twelve feet in diameter, twice the height of an average person. It is carved on one massive slab of basalt, weighs twenty-five tons, and stands in a special base for vertical display in a spacious, dramatic area at the Museum of Anthropology in Mexico City (see the following page).

The Aztec calendar is highly ordered, unlike our Gregorian calendar. Our months are uneven, and we add a day to February every four years. Nor do our months hold an even number of weeks, which makes specific dates fall on different days each year.

The Aztec calendar, on the other hand, had days, months, and years but no weeks. The Aztecs lived according to the cycle of their month, which had twenty days. Their year had eighteen months, and an extra five days—enough to make a full 365 in the year—were added and called "dead days." This was a solemn time during which all fires were extinguished, all debts were paid, and sacrifices were made for a good beginning to the new year, which was greeted with new fires, celebration, and great feasting.

The designs and information on the Aztec calendar appear in a series of concentric circles. The mathematics of the figures on the stone are complex and represent precise eras of the Aztec history of the world.

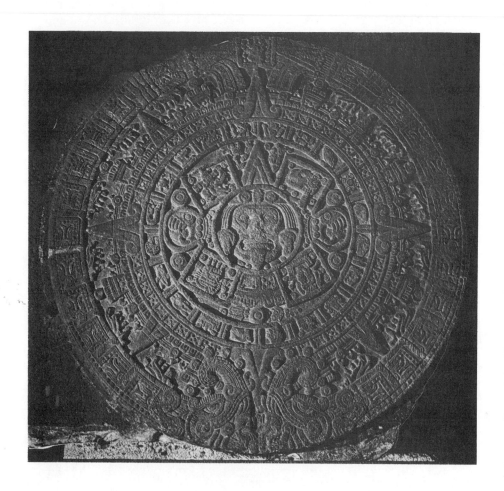

The calendar forms a series of cycles that have points of convergence, points indicating times of great religious celebrations.

At the time in history when the Great Sun Stone was carved, around 1400, Europeans believed that the earth was the center of the heavens, with the sun and stars rising and setting around it, but the Aztecs had a clear understanding that the earth revolved around the sun as part of the solar system. Building on Mayan astronomy, they accurately calculated the movements of the stars and planets. Many of their buildings had carefully engineered openings to admit bars of light for accurately marking solstices and equinoxes, which were important to their planting and harvest.

In many ways the Aztecs used their calendar the way we use ours today. They planned meetings, held different kinds of markets, and arranged social events for "next Flower" or "next Eagle" just the way we plan for "next Saturday" or "next Wednesday." They had days that were regular workdays and certain days that were holidays or celebration days.

But for the Aztecs, the days of their calendar were far more than just a measure of time. They felt that each day had a special meaning because of the god or character of that day. If we agreed to meet next Thursday, the name *Thursday* would only be a marker for that day. We would just decide to meet if it were convenient for both without also worrying about whether the god of Thursday favored the activity we had planned. But the Aztecs would look first for the day with the most favorable influences for their meeting, and then check on their personal commitments.

Each of the twenty days of the Aztec month has a glyph and a force or power. The Aztecs were careful to plan their personal worship, their social life, and their commercial ventures around the character or force of each day. Sometimes there were special feasts and festivals that superseded the normal activities of a day, but generally life followed a routine. (See the following page for a picture of the Aztec calendar [with only the days highlighted]. The days begin at the top, just to the left of the large arrow pointing north. The days read counterclockwise around the circle.)

For the Aztecs the calendar reflected the mystical connection they felt to the world around them. Mother Earth, Father Sun, and Life Rain were basic to their beliefs and central to their ideas about the crops they grew and the foods they ate. They lived close to the forces of nature and their ideas and feelings about these forces are reflected in their calendar.

But they took their beliefs one step further: They planned the specific foods they ate around the twenty days of the Aztec month. They ate foods consistent with the force or power of that day in order to gain that power or force for themselves. For instance, by eating deer meat on Day Deer, they hoped to acquire the power of alertness, or by eating rabbit meat on Day Rabbit they would gain speed. Some of the connections

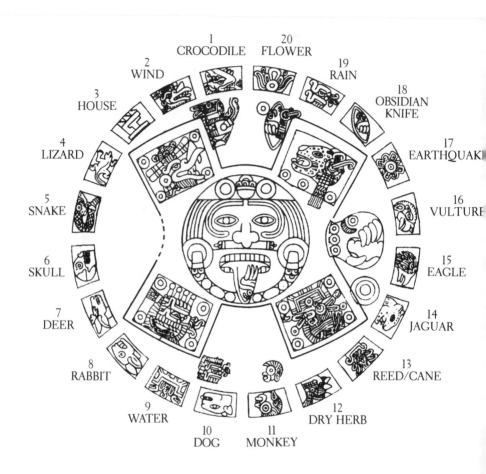

1 CROCODILE
20 FLOWER
2 WIND
19 RAIN
3 HOUSE
18 OBSIDIAN KNIFE
4 LIZARD
17 EARTHQUAKE
5 SNAKE
16 VULTURE
6 SKULL
15 EAGLE
7 DEER
14 JAGUAR
8 RABBIT
13 REED/CANE
9 WATER
12 DRY HERB
10 DOG
11 MONKEY

were as obvious as this, while others were more symbolic, such as eating fruits on Day Rain in the belief that fruits were gifts from the rain god and would refresh their bodies.

Below is a list of the calendar days, the symbols of each day, and the foods the Aztecs believed were a part of the power of that day. This is the heart of the Aztec system, their key to personal renewal, and their connection to their mystical world.

DAY	SYMBOL	POWER	FOOD
1	CROCODILE	*Quickness*	Fish
2	WIND	*Strength*	Vegetable tamales
3	HOUSE	*Love of Home*	Feast day: turkey
4	LIZARD	*Endurance*	Cactus fruit
5	SNAKE	*Meditation*	Eggs
6	SKULL	*Vitality*	Organ meats
7	DEER	*Alertness*	Deer, wild game
8	RABBIT	*Speed*	Rabbit, wild game
9	WATER	*Cleanliness*	Partial fast: fish
10	DOG	*Loyalty*	Dog
11	MONKEY	*Agility*	Fruits
12	DRY HERB	*Healing*	Vegetable/herb soups
13	REED/CANE	*Music*	Fish
14	JAGUAR	*Grace*	Feast day: turkey
15	EAGLE	*Spirituality*	Meat, beans, tortillas
16	VULTURE	*Hope*	Stewed meats
17	EARTHQUAKE	*Sensitivity*	Vegetables
18	OBSIDIAN KNIFE	*Renewal*	Cleansing fast: juice
19	RAIN	*Fertility*	Fruits
20	FLOWER	*Contentment*	Feast day: turkey, pig

3
Aztec Foods

Summer evenings, and even some days, in Mexico City are cool. It is true that Mexico City is at a tropical latitude, but it lies in a high mountain valley at an elevation of 8,000 feet. There are beautiful valleys and broad plains at every elevation down to the coast (where the climate *is* tropical, and warm to hot, all year).

These different climates make available many different kinds of foods. The Aztecs, in keeping with their industrious, inventive character, took the foods and growing methods they knew, added foods and methods acquired from the people around them, and developed an extremely productive farming system.

Their prosperity came in part from reclaiming the swamps of Lake Texcoco. They used canoes as a rapid and effective means of transportation. They dug new or wider canals where they found they needed them. To create additional farmland, they formed small islands in the broad canals they had made.

They made the islands by weaving huge mats, edged with a drawstring, to form dish shapes in the water. Then they took the dense roots and leaves of the swamp shallows and packed them into the mats and kept packing the mats until the mass reached the bottom of the swamp. They then planted willows around it to keep it from floating away. By the time the mats disintegrated, the mass was quite stable. The Aztecs would then dredge up the mud from the lake bottom and spread it on the packed vegetation, creating a soil of unrivaled richness. These islands were called *chinampas*—"floating gardens." (The modern floating gardens such as Xochimilco outside Mexico City are a small, blemished remnant of a sophisticated, effective, and highly advanced horticultural technique.)

The Aztec food staples were corn, pinto beans, several kinds of squash, and chili peppers, all of which could be dried and stored for winter use. They needed crops they could preserve to see them through the dry winter. Their climate had a distinct winter and summer, although these were denoted not by extremes of temperature but by rainy and dry seasons.

Besides the basic foods they grew, the Aztecs hunted deer, wild pig *(javalina)*, and the ducks and other wildfowl that lived in the reed marshes of the lake. They hunted the large game with bows and arrows and the smaller game with snares. They also fished the lake waters with nets and bone hooks. A wide choice of tropical plants, especially various fruits, was also an important part of their diet.

Busy trade routes and an active commerce meant that a large city like Tenochtitlán offered over a hundred products in its markets. Produce stalls offered both items grown under the ground, such as sweet potatoes, peanuts, and onions, and colorful crops cultivated above ground such as corn, beans, squash, tomatoes, melons, and jicama. These were carefully arranged in high mounds to catch the eye of the buyer, along with spices such as sage, parsley, and coriander. Easily bruised fruits such as mango, papaya, guava, and bananas were carefully spread out. Sales of fish, turkey, duck, javalina, and dog depended on the feast and season. Nonfood items such as pottery, baskets, and jewelry were also sold, along with woven lengths of cloth, fresh flowers, and bird feathers.

Barter was the basis for Aztec commerce, and the value of an item was established by desirability and availability. The cacao bean, from which chocolate is made, was a medium of exchange, as it was universally wanted and easily portable.

The marketplace buzzed with noise and activity as the vendors touted their wares and animals brought live to the market barked and called. Sweet and sour smells alternated as the aromas of fresh fruit and flowers suddenly gave way in the shifting breeze to the pungent odor of animal dung and the sour smell of discarded rinds and rotting unsold items.

Our supermarkets today feature many products found in the Aztec markets, and many foods we regularly eat now were originally cultivated or domesticated by very early tribes, added to by the Mayans and others, and then adopted by the Aztecs. Look for example, at a modern Thanksgiving Day menu and see what it would be like without Aztec foods.

THANKSGIVING MENU	NON-AZTEC FOODS
1. Turkey	1.
2. Cornbread dressing	2.
3. Cranberry sauce	3. Cranberry sauce
4. Candied sweet potatoes	4.
5. Baked squash	5.

THANKSGIVING MENU	NON-AZTEC FOODS
6. Lettuce, tomato, and avocado salad	6. Lettuce
7. Relish tray: olives, pickles, spiced apples	7. Relish tray: olives, pickles, spiced apples
8. Pumpkin pie	8.
9. After-dinner chocolate	9.

Aztec foods on this menu include: corn, turkey, members of the squash family, sweet potatoes, tomatoes, avocado, and chocolate.

Other Aztec contributions to foods we eat today are peanuts and vanilla, and tropical fruits such as banana, papaya, mango, and guava. Note, too, that the names of some Mexican foods we are familiar with actually come from the Aztec language, Nahuatl. The words have a Spanish spelling since the Spanish-speaking priests and friars were among the first to write them down. For example:

ENGLISH	SPANISH	NAHUATL (AZTEC)
Avocado	Aguacate	Aguacatl
Tamale	Tamale	Tamal
Pinto Beans	Frijoles	Frijol
Turkey	Guajolote	Guajolotl
Chocolate	Chocolate	Chocolatl
Tomato	Tomate	Tomatl

The great variety of nutritious foods that originated on this continent was a key factor in the vitality of the Aztec people. Proof of the benefits of the Aztec life-style is the stark contrast to life in Europe at the same time.

In Europe bathing was rare. The hands preparing food to be eaten were often unclean, going from tending animals and personal needs to the food with no washing in between. Dysentery, parasites, worms, many fevers, and other ailments were common. Grossly unsanitary conditions and practices made plagues a constant threat. With no refrigeration available, foods spoiled quickly but were eaten anyway. Foods not eaten one day were often saved for the next, especially in times of want, despite discolorations and bad odors. Cooking and serving utensils were not well-cleaned.

For the Aztecs, on the other hand, bathing was a ritual and personal necessity. Their religion fostered washing, and the hands preparing the food were usually clean. The Aztecs cooked and prepared foods so that there was little spoilage. Broiling over coals—a clean way to prepare foods—was a popular cooking method for many meats. Plant husks such as corn and banana leaves were commonly used to hold foods to be cooked and were placed in a bed of coals. They were discarded after one use, avoiding the problem of bacteria growth on poorly washed utensils. Outdoor ovens were used as well, and they reached a temperature high enough to keep baked foods (cooked in pottery and stone dishes) hot until they were served.

Because each day had its own distinctive main meal, many foods, especially meat dishes, were not saved from one day to the next. Cooks were careful with ingredient amounts, and leftovers were given to the dogs and the turkeys.

Until the Spanish brought respiratory ailments, there were no plagues or sweeping epidemics among the Aztecs, and the people lived well and long. Colds, smallpox, measles, and chickenpox were devastating to them, for they had no immunity to these diseases (the devastation from these plagues is documented in the *Codex Florentino*), and they died by the thousands. Anthropologists estimate that half the population of Tenochtitlán died within the first few years of contact with the Spaniards. Until then they were generally healthy and felt they were partaking of the universe's great and desirable powers as they ate the different foods assigned to each of the twenty days of their calendar.

Aztec and Modern Mexican-American Foods

As we consider the foods included in the Aztec diet, it is important to distinguish them from "Mexican" foods.

Mexican food is popular in the United States, with its unique tastes and satisfying portions. However, this Mexican food does *not* resemble Aztec food (or even much of the food actually eaten in Mexico today). Mexican dishes have some Aztec ingredients, but there the similarity ends. They differ from Aztec foods in four crucial ways:

1. Mexican food in the U.S. is increasingly deep-fried to appeal to the North American palate, and even foods that aren't fried are prepared with a considerable amount of oil. The Aztecs rarely used frying as a cooking method. They braised over coals, stewed, simmered, baked, and used a stone griddle. Fats were seldom used because they quickly turned rancid in the tropics.

2. There is a trend away from baked corn tortillas to deep-fried flour tortillas. The Aztecs did have a white flour (from the amaranth plant), but it was not made into tortillas, and their tortillas were not fried.

3. Mexican foods use cheese. The Aztecs did not have cheese since they had no goats or cows.

4. Mexican foods use ground or sliced beef, whereas the Aztecs did not have beef.

Fats, white flour, cheese, and beef: None of the contemporary "Mexican" culprits were to be found in the healthful, life-invigorating foods of the Aztecs.

4
Nutrition

The young girls heartily detested the old woman who called herself Crested Bird. They called her Worm Bird, implying not that she ate worms but that her body was made of worms.

Crested Bird had built herself a reputation as a fine teacher. Those who had managed to make it through her unyielding tutelage in cooking appreciated the skills they'd acquired, and some even professed a grudging affection for her. The young girls in her current flock did not believe a word of it, for they had to face her pride every day. That hers was an earned pride made it no easier to bear. She never tired of telling them of the day one of the Great High Priests had come to her home. He wanted to make sure that her teaching of the Sun Stone principles was correct. Taking advantage of the Aztec respect for teachers, especially old women, she had not lain on the floor as most of her station would have done; she had merely knelt, not even bowing her head.

"He came with the governor of my district," Crested Bird would say to the girls. "As the governor gasped at my seeming lack of respect, I turned to him and told him that a true noble respects knowledge and teaching in whomever he finds it." She would invariably give an odd shrug of her right shoulder as she said these words, which the girls derisively pantomimed when they were alone in their sleeping hut adjacent to Crested Bird's house. "The noble honored that statement and even extended his hand that I might rise and stand at his level," she would add. Then, like her namesake, Crested Bird would slowly draw her head down, as though displaying an imaginary crest of brilliant feathers.

She had the girls up before dawn every day, insisting on a thorough washing ritual from each. "A dirty, itchy body turns away understanding" was one of her oft-quoted sayings. She was kind to those who were genuinely ill, but she had an uncanny ability to know when one of her flock was feigning some malady to avoid getting up. The consequences were swift and sure. Grasping the girl by her hair, she would pull her off her sleeping mat, roll up the mat, order the girl to gather what few belongings might be hers, and send her home. The girl would then face serious punishment from her family, who would be ashamed that their daughter was thus dispatched.

All of Crested Bird's teachings were from oral tradition. Those with a talent for learning what they heard gained ready praise from the teacher, while those who would have been quick to grasp any picture or drawing or visual representation did not fare as well.

Each morning's teaching ritual was the same. The girls would be on their mats lined along the veranda, a shawl or rug under them as they would first kneel, then sit back on their heels, then move their feet to the sides to suit the comfort of each girl. In front of each girl was a rectangular stone about two feet long and one foot wide, hollowed in the center in a smooth crescent. With it was a heavy cylindrical stone eight or nine inches long, rounded to an oval shape at each end. These were each girl's most basic tools; with them she would grind corn for *maza*, the dough for forming tortillas, the basic staple of Aztec life.

"Today *iiiiis*," Crested Bird would begin, drawing out the last word in a long singsong that would start her rhythm of questions and answers. On cue the girls would respond in chorus, giving the day's date. On the first day of the new year, they would say "One Crocodile." Twenty-one days later they would say "Two Crocodile," and twenty-one days after that "Three Crocodile," until each of the twenty days had been named eighteen times in numerical sequence.

This day the answer was "Seven Monkey." Crested Bird's eyes moved quickly from face to face as she listened for a lag in the answer that would show that a girl was echoing instead of knowing.

Without pause or praise, the singsong continued. "The power of today *iiiiis*," and on cue the answer came: "Agility."

"The source of the power?"

"Fruits."

"The source of the fruits?"

"Tlaloc." [The rain god.]

"The kind of food?"

"Sweet, with the wetness of the rain. A gift, from above the ground."

"And it strengthens?"

"The body first and the spirit second."

Again there was no praise, the reward of correct answers being that no one was called upon singly and taunted before the group for her display of ignorance. The only reaction from the teacher was a nod and a short "Hmmm."

"Now, quickly to the corn!"

The girls rose as a body and filed past a mat where kernels of corn had been neatly piled. The corn had been boiled in a weak solution of calcium carbonate (water with limestone added), and its hulls were clean and soft. Each took as much corn as she could scoop in both hands and, placing it next to the long grinding stone, knelt again. This time the girls did not sit back on their heels. They took half of their corn and placed it in the hollow of the long stone. Then they took the cylindrical stone and, using the weight of their upper bodies, began quickly to grind the golden kernels. Deftly they gathered the first coarse grindings and added new kernels under the hand stone and reworked them until there was a smooth, pale-yellow mound of dough at the bottom of the stone.

Now, taking a ball of dough about the size of her palm, each girl would pat and clap it into an even circle of dough about ten inches in diameter. Crested Bird had a way of using the heel of her right hand against the palm of her left to create an especially smooth tortilla and the girls earnestly tried to copy her, but she was so skilled and deft it was hard to follow the sequence of her moves.

Each girl then held up her tortilla in both hands while Crested Bird examined her work. Crested Bird was harsh, but she was fair. If the tortilla was perfectly rounded and perfectly even, she let it pass. If not, a salvo of criticism ensued.

In the patio, Crested Bird's maid began adding kindling to a small fire under a thin slab of sandstone, the cooking surface for the tortillas. The girls began to grow restless, hungry for the tortillas they had just made, hoping their teacher would be brief.

In her mind Crested Bird heard the repeated rhythm of the days of the calendar and their sources, and they seemed to her like a woven braid, alternating foods for physical strength with foods for spiritual strength. Crested Bird explained this dimension to her flock. Some could hear the rhythm of the alternation around the circle of the calendar that others could not. Still, all of the girls were concerned about making sure that, when asked, they could recite the twenty days and their powers in correct order. At night when they lay upon their sleeping mats, they would whisper the round of the calendar endlessly to one another, naming the day, its power, and its main food until they drifted to sleep.

"The hungry care not for music," said Crested Bird loudly. The girls nodded and watched Crested Bird mentally congratulate herself on another of her profound sayings. It was important to nod solemnly even if they weren't sure what it meant.

"Would you tell us more about that?" asked one of the girls. Crested Bird was delighted to expound, even though the question had been asked more to flatter her than to gain real information.

"Some powers give strength to the spirit. If one of you has had no food for three days, and your friend says that she will help you, and then she sings you a song, she has not helped you at all! Even"—and here Crested Bird paused dramatically—"if it is a song about Quetzalcoatl!" Visualizing Quetzalcoatl, the Plumed Serpent, one of the Aztecs' main deities, the girls nodded again, but this time in quick nods of understanding.

Taking the hand of the girl nearest her and pointing to the network of scars crisscrossing the pads of the girl's fingers, Crested Bird continued: "If you cut your fingers for the blood of sacrifice and place it in an offering stone but see only blood, feel only useless pain, then you have wasted your effort! If you stuff your mouth hurriedly to quiet your stomach, there is no room for spirit. You see only blood, you eat only food, and soon you have no strength, for you have forgotten that your blood represents the vitality of your spirit, which you give, and that the food represents the vitality of all the spirits, which you receive!"

The girls tried to look as though they always saw the vitality, although some had never felt that inspiration, and for most it was only an occasional experience.

"So!" continued Crested Bird, "You must receive some powers that feed the spirit, and some powers that feed the body. They come from spirits that live in the water, and some that live on the land, and some that grow from rain, and some that arise from toil. And they must come next to each other in a certain way, so that there is first one of one kind and one of another!"

Crested Bird was now engrossed in her subject, walking back and forth in front of the girls and gesturing widely and eloquently as she spoke of one spiritual force and then another. The girls sat in obedient silence, their eyes dutifully fixed on their teacher's face, trying to understand her words and trying to ignore their hunger.

The tall figure of one of the governor's aides moved slowly into the room. Crested Bird was pleased she had been found expounding so forcefully, for she knew full well that this scene would be carefully reported to the governor. She bowed very low, and all the girls touched their foreheads to the ground in front of them, grateful for this reprieve.

Although few of today's teachers use tactics quite so severe, we are no less careful to teach our children about the importance of eating the right foods. Education in the four food groups is a standard component in the health curriculum of our primary schools. We strive for nutritional balance with care and knowledge, as did the Aztecs.

For the Aztecs, a *day* was their typical nutrition unit. For us, a balanced *meal* is a common measure of good nutrition. Nutritionists today are moving away from a balanced meal toward a balanced *diet*, but much of what is still taught in school centers around a balanced meal, and children are taught to look for the "basic four" in a meal.

Twenty days, which is what the Aztecs had, provides a framework for the rotation of foods. The Aztecs had several factors in their rotation, going from feast to fast, meat to nonmeat, and days of emphasis on vegetables or days of emphasis on fruits.

Balance of the Twenty Days

Within the twenty days of their calendar, the Aztecs balanced contrasting forces or powers gained from the food and ruling spirit of each day. The powers gained were either for spiritual well-being or physical well-being, although it is a little arbitrary to divide them since, then as now, each is supported by the other. It is difficult to feel spiritual when the body is suffering, and the body is without total vigor when the spirit is suffering. The Aztecs felt that a sickly, malnourished body did not have the strength to accept the powers of each day. They also felt that a strong body, no matter how well-trained, was of little benefit if the person had no spiritual goals to provide motivation and joy for living. They felt that the rhythmic repetition of a large variety of foods provided value, strength, and force to food utilization. The calendar itself provided the balance they sought.

Features of the Twenty Days

The twenty days are divided along two axes. The first is the north–south line through the calendar (see page 26). The days and powers the Aztecs associated with each day are then divided equally.

There are ten days in each half of the calendar. Within each of the ten days are five days that give physical powers and four days that give spiritual powers. There is also a day of fasting in each half, one at day number nine and one at day number eighteen.

The days alternate so that there are never more than two consecutive days of either physical or spiritual powers.

The kinds of foods eaten on each of the calendar days are also balanced. The Aztecs considered meat dishes to be one kind of food, non-meat dishes to be another kind of food, with vegetables grown below ground having a different source of power than those grown above ground. This latter distinction came from the fact that foods grown above the ground—such as golden corn, bright red peppers, rosy mangoes, variegated squash—often have the bright colors of the sun. Foods grown below ground are often white or beige (potatoes, cassava, or peanuts) or orange (carrots and sweet potatoes), the rich colors of the earth.

Following the north–south division, the kinds of foods the Aztecs associated with each day are also in balance. The first ten-day group has six days of animal-source dishes, three days of plant-source dishes, and one partial-fast day. The second group has five days of animal-source dishes, four days of plant-source dishes, and one juice-fast day (see page 27).

Adding the east–west axis to segment the calendar into quarters, the pattern of powers in each quadrant is again balanced (see page 29).

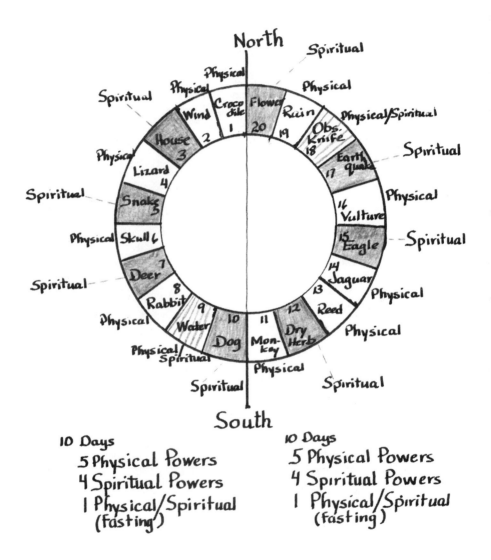

North

South

10 Days
5 Physical Powers
4 Spiritual Powers
1 Physical/Spiritual
(fasting)

10 Days
5 Physical Powers
4 Spiritual Powers
1 Physical/Spiritual
(fasting)

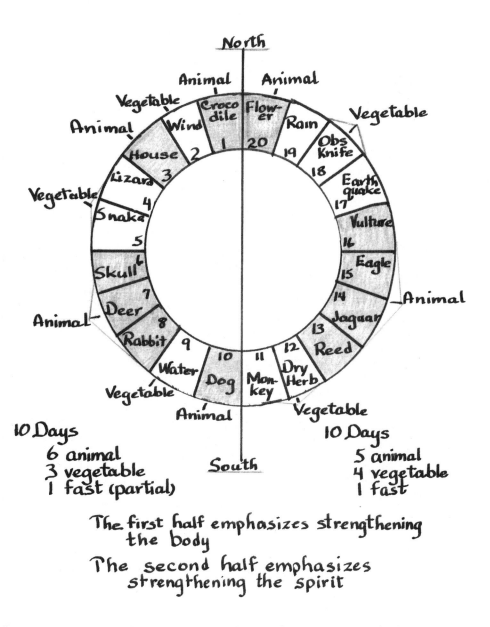

North

Animal

Animal

Vegetable

Animal

Vegetable

Animal

Vegetable

Vegetable

Animal

Animal

Vegetable

Animal

Vegetable

Wind 2 1 Croco-dile	Flow-er 20	Rain 19
House 3		Obs knife 18
Lizard 4		Earth quake 17
Snake 5		Vulture 16
Skull 6 7		Eagle 15
Deer 8		14
Rabbit 9		Jaguar 13
Water 10	Dog	Reed 12
	Monkey 11	Dry Herb

South

10 Days
6 animal
3 vegetable
1 fast (partial)

10 Days
5 animal
4 vegetable
1 fast

The first half emphasizes strengthening
the body

The second half emphasizes
strengthening the spirit

NW   3 physical powers
     2 spiritual powers

SW   2 physical powers
     2 spiritual powers
     1 fast (physical-spiritual powers)

SE   3 physical powers
     2 spiritual powers

NE   2 physical powers
     2 spiritual powers
     1 fast (physical-spiritual powers)

Crested Bird had her platitudes, and so do we, including "The times they are a-changin'." And those changing times are especially apparent in our food-processing and food-consumption patterns. Once everything was laboriously prepared by hand in the home. Mealtimes were important "family" times of day. Today technological and social changes have made meals an eat-when-you-can event. Daily family gatherings for mother's home cooking are more and more rare. Many foods are partially or completely processed. Frequent meals at fast-food and other restaurants have increased fat, salt, and calorie consumption, often to the detriment of the consumer's health.

The fact that you have this book in your hands suggests that you care about healthy nutrition for yourself and those who share their lives with you, that you are intellectually open, and that you are able to make commitments to matters that are important. You delight in things that are fine, and you have a sparkle of innovation and the ability to take the "ordinary" and see its potential for humor, drama, or fun. In terms of food, it means you will probably enjoy the kinds of foods the Aztecs ate and will understand the connections they made to the world as they saw it. They felt that different kinds of foods could give different kinds of energy, beliefs that are fully described for each of the twenty days.

Technology today gives us the ability to analyze our foods at the molecular level. Because of these marvelous chemical and medical tools, we have precise knowledge of why particular kinds of foods are good for our bodies.

The Aztecs had a solid body of knowledge also, based on observing the results of eating certain foods. They did not know *why* certain combinations of foods were beneficial, but they were aware of these combinations. They tied that knowledge to their profound spiritual connection with the universe, believing that their gods gave certain powers to their foods. Though it involves their beliefs, their system of nutrition, placed in a time unit broader than one day, is valid and has most of the elements

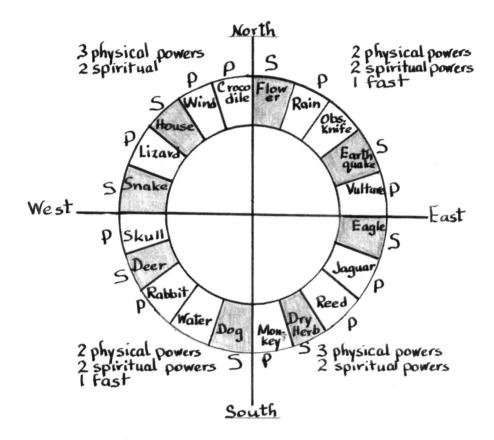

we have been fortunate enough to make part of our general knowledge of nutrition.

The Aztecs classified foods according to their source and the kind of life force they represented. We categorize foods according to their nutritional content. The end results in terms of balancing foods to give the body optimum nutrition are amazingly similar, for each system provides for a variety of foods to be used in certain combinations that nourish the body in a healthy way.

The Modern Food Groups

Today's foods are often divided into four groups on the basis of nutrient content. Our traditional notion of an ideal meal contains servings from at least three of these groups.

1. **Protein:** meats, nuts, eggs, legumes (beans, lentils, soybeans); 2 SMALL SERVINGS DAILY ARE RECOMMENDED

2. **Dairy:** milk and milk products such as cheese, ice cream, yogurt; 2 SERVINGS DAILY

3. **Grains:** breads, pasta products, cereals; 4 SERVINGS DAILY

4. **Fruits and Vegetables:** dark-green, leafy or orange vegetables, and fruits, including 1 citrus fruit; 4 SERVINGS DAILY

The Aztec Food Groups

Aztec foods were also placed into four basic food groups, but were categorized by source and effect on the body:

1. **Mother Earth plus cultivation:** agricultural products such as beans, corn, and squash.
   Effect: Give strength of Mother Earth.

2. **Rain:** fruits, especially juicy, tropical ones.
   Effect: Refresh and cleanse.

3. **Water dwellers:** fish, other water animals such as crab, octopus, alligator, and turtle.
   Effect: Give strength to digestion.

4. **Animal:** deer, rabbit, turkey, wild pig, and the like.
   Effect: Give spark of vitality.

Their ideal *day* contained foods from each of the first two sources and one from either group 3 or group 4.

The Aztec system had two advantages. The first was that the calendar provided a framework of great order that was long enough—twenty days —to avoid boring repetition. The second was the psychological factor that each day had significant emotional and spiritual meaning.

Today's fundamentals of proper nutrition include the following as essential nutrients:

1. **Protein** Every cell in the body contains protein. Proteins make up the chief solid matter of muscles, organs, and endocrine glands. They are the building blocks for bones and teeth, and are the main components of the cells that form skin, nails, and hair. Proteins build the cells that make up our blood and the antibodies that provide resistance to disease. Protein provides for growth and the maintenance of body tissues.

Proteins are made up of amino acids—twenty-two different amino acids in a complete protein. The body can produce many of these to meet its own needs, but there are nine the body cannot produce, and these nine must be provided by specific foods. Meats contain all twenty-two amino acids, but are not the only sources of protein. Nutritionists speak of protein complementarity, in which foods are specifically combined to guarantee that all twenty-two amino acids are present for nutritional use.

2. **Carbohydrates** Carbohydrates, formed of carbon and hydrogen and oxygen, are the most abundant organic compounds in our world. They are the energy that plants store as sugars through photosynthesis.

Carbohydrates are readily digested and provide a main energy source for the body. They are changed easily into blood sugar (glucose), the prime body fuel for the brain and muscles as well as other body tissues. Carbohydrates are the body's preferred source of energy, saving the proteins for tissue-building and repair. Should a shortage of carbohydrates require it, the body will convert fat and protein to carbohydrates, but that chemical process can put a significant strain on the kidneys.

Complex carbohydrates in whole grains, breads, and potatoes have a beneficial effect on the body for energy and also contribute other important nutrients, such as B-complex vitamins. Carbohydrates taken as sugars, candies, pastries, and cake/cookie items are sometimes eaten in place of more nutritional foods, which may affect the body adversely.

3. **Fats** Fats, or lipids, are a concentrated form of energy. They have a greasy feel and do not dissolve in water. They are made up of fatty acids and glycerol, whose various combinations determine how hard a fat is, what its melting point is, and how quickly it oxidizes or turns rancid.

With our current concern about the high proportion of fats in our diet, it is easy to overlook the fact that the body needs fats to function properly. They are such a concentrated source of energy that even small amounts of fats represent large amounts of calories, a fact well known by calorie-conscious people. However, fats should not be totally eliminated from the diet. They are needed to deliver the fat-soluble vitamins (A, D, E, and K) to all parts of the body and to promote the efficient functioning of nerve and hormonal mechanisms. Cholesterol is a necessary body component and is synthesized and regulated by the liver. Problems with cholesterol usually stem from excessive consumption of this vital nutrient.

Saturated fats are derived from animal fats and dairy products and some plants, such as coconuts. Commercially hydrogenated shortenings and the animal and dairy fats are solid at room temperature. These tend to raise the amount of cholesterol in the blood.

Unsaturated or *polyunsaturated fats* are usually derived from vegetable oils, such as corn or safflower, or nuts, such as almonds. They are liquid at room temperature and tend to lower cholesterol levels.

4. **Vitamins** Vitamins are essential to the enzyme systems that allow the body to absorb and use amino acids, carbohydrates, and fats. They are usually classified in two major groups: the water-soluble group, the B vitamins and vitamin C; and the fat-soluble group, vitamins A, D, E, and K.

Vitamins were studied and identified in response to diseases or disorders that could be cured with the addition of specific nutrients in the diet. These findings established their vital role in maintaining good health, but opened debates that continue today as to whether supplements may be needed.

5. **Minerals** Minerals are part of the structure of every cell of the body. The amount of a mineral present in the body is not related to its importance. Even a few milligrams of some minerals can make the difference between health and deficiency. Minerals help regulate the permeability of cell membranes, the contraction of muscles, and the response of nerves to stimuli and play a part in maintaining the equilibrium of acids and bases in the body.

6. **Water** Water is second only to oxygen as a vital body requirement. A person can live for several weeks without food but for only a few days without water. Even a loss of 10 percent of the body's water is a serious health hazard, because water is the medium of all body fluids—the digestive juices, blood, urine, and perspiration. Water is a basic component of all cells.

Water is essential for digestion: Food products are turned into a watery mixture in the intestine so they can be absorbed through the intestinal walls into the bloodstream. Water carries these nutrients to the body cells and takes wastes to kidneys and lower intestine for disposal.

Water regulates body temperature. Water carries the heat generated by the cells and distributes it throughout the body, and perspiration, forming on the skin, cools by evaporation.

Adequate amounts of water promote healthy kidney and colon function. Hair, nails, and skin are dependent on water to stay healthy and flexible rather than brittle and, in the case of the skin, to stay elastic and less apt to dry and wrinkle.

The Aztecs did not have this body of detailed information, but they used careful observation to achieve their excellent food balance. That process was not unique to the Aztecs, of course; similar systems were employed independently by the Chinese, Romans, and Egyptians with documented success. The Aztecs' observations were probably similar to those that led to the discovery of vitamins, finding that certain diseases and disorders could be cured by adding certain foods to the diet. And their observations led to a foodstyle that provided them a healthy lifestyle.

1. **Protein** The Aztecs included a variety of animal sources for protein and guaranteed it in their basic food items of beans and corn, which were always served together. These two foods are a legume and a grain, respectively, which combine to form a complete protein. The Aztecs did not typically consume large amounts of meat, even on days when a meat was the staple of that day's menu, but this was not a detriment to good nutrition. When plant-food protein is mixed with even a small amount of animal protein, the result is as nutritionally effective as if only animal sources for protein had been used.

2. **Carbohydrates** Whole grains and cereals are the staple sources of carbohydrates, and the ground corn of tortillas and tamales provided a daily source of this nutrient for the Aztecs. The beans the Aztecs ate not only provided protein, they were also a significant source of carbohydrates, yielding around 60 grams of carbohydrate for every 100 grams of dry, uncooked beans. The complex starches found in fruits, vegetables, and sources such as nuts and certain root plants were also excellent carbohydrate sources, especially in their natural, unrefined state. The Aztecs also used honey, in which 80 percent of the weight is carbohydrates (the other 20 percent is water) and 100 percent of the calories are from carbohydrates.

3. **Fats** The Aztecs' extensive use of corn provided generous amounts of polyunsaturated fats. Peanuts, sunflower seeds, pumpkin seeds, and avocados, which were also important foods commonly used by the Aztecs, provided additional daily sources of fats in the diet. These were supplemented by the fats in the meats that they ate.

4. **Vitamins** The foods eaten by the Aztecs contained many vitamins with which we are now familiar. Just as we receive a variety of vitamins by eating many different foods, both cooked and raw, so did the Aztecs.

5. **Minerals** The Aztecs did not have any of the nutritional supplements that are available to us today but, judging from the health they enjoyed, we can assume that the soils in which they grew their crops were rich and provided most of the minerals essential for good health. In the area around Tenochtitlán, farm areas were created in the lake itself through land-forming techniques that used the equivalent of compost, which is rich in natural nutrients. Volcanic soils, which were the kinds of soils most available for farming, are also rich in minerals.

5. **Water** Water was a revered element to the Aztecs. They were aware of its vital need by the body, and it was taken freely throughout the day. Juices were seen as related to water, and offering juice to a guest entering a home was standard Aztec courtesy. The habitual drinking of Morning Rain (which offers the body liquids instead of food) first thing in the morning was very beneficial to health; this was a daily practice, not a ritual or occasional custom.

By any standard, the foods of the Aztec calendar provided excellent nutrition. Broad guidelines for a balanced diet suggest that each day include:

Proteins:	provided by meats or legume/grain foods
Vitamin C:	provided by tomatoes, mangoes, papayas, melons, chilies
Vitamin A:	provided by mangoes, papayas, sweet potatoes, squash, tomatoes, and corn
Carbohydrates:	provided by corn, beans, amaranth, jicama, bananas, coconut, fruits
Fats:	provided by fats in meats, peanuts, corn
Minerals and Vitamins:	provided by vegetables and fruits, whole grains, beans, and meat

Each of these categories is represented in each of the eighteen food days in the calendar. An exception is calcium. The Aztecs prepared their dried corn kernels in limestone water, which contains calcium carbonate. (Forensic studies of Aztec skeletons show sound teeth and bones, so apparently their application and use of lime provided adequate amounts of this important mineral.) Our milling processes today do not do this, so a calcium supplement is sometimes suggested. To this the Aztecs added fasting, which they used to give the body a time to rest and be cleansed.

The Aztecs left us a rich legacy of knowledge about foods that fit our needs today. The American Heart Association and the American Cancer Society are two organizations that have published dietary recommendations based on research. Their conclusions are that low-fiber, high-fat foods and empty calories are current obstacles to good health.

The American Heart Association recommends the reduction of dietary fat and cholesterol intake. The menus suggested in the Aztec diet contain only small amounts of fat and cholesterol. Since the Aztecs did not fry their foods, the cholesterol is present in the animal foods and eggs, as well as smaller amounts in such plant foods as peanuts or avocados. They did not use oil or butter sauces, which is where many hidden calories and fats show up in our diet today. The vegetables are not served with oil or any sauce, and the grain foods (tortillas and Aztec muffins), are served with honey, not margarine or butter.

The Aztec diet is low in red meat. Their main red meats were venison, dog, and javelina (wild pig). Lamb, substituted for dog in this food plan, leaves a total of only three days of red meat in the total of twenty days. The diet is low in meat consumption in general—eleven of twenty days —yet proteins are generously supplied.

The World Health Organization is charged with the task of searching for adequate protein levels in poor countries and countries where meat is prohibited on religious grounds. Their research suggests that a diet in which protein comes from plants as well as from animal sources may, in fact, be much better for overall health than one in which meat consumed every day satisfies the protein requirement. The Aztec diet, which furnishes complete proteins by combining legumes and grains as well as from animal sources, is perfectly suited for that need.

The American Cancer Society emphasizes the need for natural fiber sources and inclusion of key vegetables in the diet, especially dark-green and orange vegetables, which are important in cancer prevention. These important foods are well represented in the Aztec diet.

The Aztec diet is also quite high in natural fiber, since fruits and vegetables are the main ingredients of the morning and evening meals. The Aztecs considered these foods a vital and important part of their daily diet, not an addendum to satisfy the need to have three or four food groups represented in one meal. (Or what you had to eat in order to get dessert!) Many foods in the Aztec diet provide natural fiber, especially avocados, beans, carrots, coconuts, guavas, nuts, onions, and sweet peppers.

Fruits and vegetables are the main source of many vitamins and minerals. In general, the citrus fruits are high in vitamin C, as are mangoes, papayas, chili peppers, and some dark-green vegetables such as broccoli.

The orange-colored vegetables like carrots and squash provide vitamin A in its natural, beneficial form of beta carotene.

The Aztec diet is basically lactose-free. The Aztecs had no dairy animals, and so milk as a beverage as well as its many derivatives are not a part of this food system. In some recipes in this book, cream cheese is nevertheless listed as an ingredient. To provide a lactose-free diet, substitutions are given. Also, other cheese-free Aztec recipes could be substituted for these dishes.

The Aztec diet is a boon to anyone who needs to be on a wheat-free diet. As you look at the menus suggested for each day, you will see that some have muffins or rolls, particularly at snack time, but these are not integral to the system. The only other recipe that uses wheat is the Sweet Pockets recipe on page 166, which has a wheat dough shell. By eliminating that one recipe and by substituting tortillas for the occasions that have the muffins or rolls, you have a complete and satisfying foodstyle with corn rather than wheat as its base.

Because of the different character of each day of the Aztec calendar, and because the foods alternate from day to day, the foods balance each other in nutrient content. It is very difficult, using a variety of foods as the source of nutrients, to become seriously out of balance. Eating large quantities of any particular food goes against anything suggested in the meal pattern of the Sun Stone—and against your own common sense.

To the Aztecs, their foods were not a diet, they were their way of life. They knew times of want, which made times of plenty all the more appreciated. Their foods were intimately associated with their worship and their beliefs of how the elements of their world nourished them and how they were to receive these vital gifts from their gods. To them, the powers they associated with the different foods were their keys to health and energy. The combined powers and foods nourished both spirit and body, and provided a binding link to their world and culture.

5
Adapting the Aztec Foodstyle for Today

The Aztecs believed in their food system because it was tied to the influence of the gods or characters of their calendar. For example, when they ate the rabbit called for on Day Rabbit, they would think about speed. They would imagine themselves as having greater speed. Because they were visualizing speed and focusing on it they probably did, in fact, walk or run more quickly. This affirmed their belief that eating rabbit on its designated day proved effective.

The Aztec food system works for us because it is so complete. Their rules for the use and combining of foods are so nutritionally sound that we can take advantage of their food system without believing in their pantheon. At the same time, we can enjoy learning about the connections they made between their natural and supernatural worlds.

There is power and vitality in what the Aztecs learned and used. For you to make use of this information in your life, I have taken this research and put it into a *menu format*. The glyph or picture that appears on the calendar for that day is shown, along with couplets reflecting the spiritual inspiration the Aztecs saw in that day. I have then included a commentary on that spirit, or the Aztec way of celebrating that spirit, and the principal food that goes with it. Next is the menu for that day, with page numbers where each recipe is found, followed by nutritional information on the foods for that day.

As they developed this system Aztec healers and priests looked for the foods and combinations that were effective. They felt they were looking for the activities and foods that were pleasing to their gods. When people felt energetic and healthy, then they must, in their beliefs, be properly obedient. The Aztecs produced a very detailed system for using foods to promote their health and longevity.

The first result of this system is a sequence of foods that is balanced, containing complete protein on most days, yet very low in fats. It includes a variety of fruits and vegetables and plenty of natural fiber.

The second result is that the Aztec system, with its abundance of energy-giving foods and low fat, has the effect of moderating weight. The effects are nothing like a sudden or crash loss of weight, which is usually temporary and sometimes even unhealthy because it may force the body to draw energy from vital organs when food intake is suddenly lowered. Fad diets sometimes rely on the overuse of one particular food or food substitute, which does not give the body time to change its metabolism rate slowly. Listlessness and irritability often accompany these rapid changes. When the restrictions end, the body regains the lost weight. With the Aztec diet the body remains well-nourished while excess pounds are lost in a slow and consistent way.

As you use the Aztec foods, there are four differences from our current life-style to keep in mind.

Separation of Foods

The Aztecs kept certain foods separate. Fruits and vegetables, for example, were not eaten at the same meal. They were seen to have opposing natures that belonged to different times of the day. In general, fruits were associated with the rain god and were considered gifts, probably because of their generally juicy quality and the fact that they were often harvested from trees that grew naturally. Even when farmed, they did not require laborious cultivation. Fruits and their juices were taken in the morning to refresh the body the way rain refreshes the earth.

Vegetables were the staples of the Aztec diet. Corn, pinto beans, and squash were considered the strength of life. They are watered twice: once by rain or irrigation and then by the sweat of effort that goes into their cultivation. Given vitality by Father Sun and Mother Earth, these foods were served midday and evening.

The Time of Day of Meals

The famous Mexican siesta—the long afternoon rest—is a strong Aztec tradition. Food was prepared in the cooler morning time and the main meal was eaten in the middle of the day. This was followed by a siesta, and activities resumed in the late afternoon and continued into early evening. A light meal was taken at night. This was an ideal plan for living in comfort in the tropic regions of the Aztec empire. It also kept the body from having to cope with its heaviest load of digestion during the long inactivity of nighttime sleep.

Since most of us do not live in the tropics, our culture does not foster this schedule. Should you have some time flexibility, however, you would enjoy trying this, because it does benefit the body.

Separation of Food and Drink

The Aztecs drank juices and water freely throughout the day but did not serve water or juice with their food. At certain feast-day banquets a cacao-bean beverage and *pulque*, a potent alcoholic drink, were served, but they were tied to ritual and were not the daily custom.

Morning Rain

Morning Rain is taken on first arising, at least half an hour before any other food. This is a vital part of the Aztec system. It is made by taking ¼ glass of any kind of juice and ¾ glass of warm or tepid water. (Remember, the Aztecs did not have any refrigeration.) For the comfort of your digestion, adhere to the warm or tepid rule. Drink 12 to 16 ounces daily, whatever the other foods of the day might be.

The Aztecs' diet, combined with their beliefs, created a way of life that was very successful. They ate foods that were vital and nourishing, and they ate a great variety of foods. They compensated for natural spoilage by having one kind of food each day and planning for few leftovers. They had great energy and stamina, and felt prepared to meet the challenges of everyday life.

We wish for energy and stamina also and are aware that it is best gotten from foods that are low in fat, low in cholesterol, and high in fiber. Many people also need foods that are wheat-free and milk-free. Those very important benefits characterize the Aztec Way. To their foods the Aztecs then added their profound, mystical appreciation for the life force within those foods, bringing a dimension of joy to the important act of eating.

About the Menus

The menus in this book are not directly from any original Aztec writings. They do follow the sequence of the Aztec calendar and use the foods and cooking styles of the Aztecs.

Adaptations to our foods and our life-style today have been made as seems sensible. In my kitchen I have a modern stove with an oven, so I don't need to bury husk-wrapped foods in coals. As I experimented with a particular dish I could then recommend an approximate size of baking dish and an oven setting. I also have a microwave oven, a wonderful, quick way to heat a stack of tortillas. I also have canned chilies and some chili powder a friend sent me from New Mexico, luxuries unknown to the Aztecs. It seems as practical to me to use today's conveniences to fix Aztec foods as any other foods. I feel that the value of the Aztec diet lies in the way the Aztec foods follow the Aztec calendar, not in having Aztec utensils or outdoor ovens. As you make substitutions of your own, try to keep to the kind of food suggested for each day in order to preserve the balance and rotation of the calendar.

The Aztecs were careful and appreciative of food and gave their choices thought and meaning. These menus keep the Aztec spirit of care and meaning.

This series of menus is intended to be flexible. The Aztecs had to allow for season and availability and certainly made substitutions and modifications. You will certainly enjoy a flexible approach also, but you do need to stay within these guidelines.

1. The Aztecs did not have cattle or goats and so did not have cheese. They did have a fermented bean curd; in the recipes here, cream cheese was suggested as a substitute where appropriate.

2. The Aztecs did not have wheat, but they produced an exceptionally nutritious flour from a plant called amaranth. Amaranth is available today in most health food stores. Whole wheat flour, preferably organic, is a good substitute.

3. You can prepare tortillas in a number of ways. Usually they are served warm in a stack and can be rolled up with honey or a jam or jelly spread on them. A microwave is a good way to heat them. Cover with either plastic or paper towel and heat for twenty to thirty seconds. (In a plastic sack, very moist, the tortillas will almost disintegrate, in a paper towel, they will be drier.)

4. The suggested midmorning snack does not include coffee. The Aztecs did not have coffee, but they did have several hot drinks made by steeping grains and various herb leaves. Herbal teas would be good modern substitutes. Although the Aztecs did not fix their hot chocolate the way we do, it is included as a possible midmorning beverage.

5. The Aztecs ate dog, which is not acceptable to us. Lamb has been substituted on the menu for the day of Dog since it is a red meat with a mild flavor.

6. Today we recognize the importance of calcium for bone and tooth structure as well as other body functions. The Aztec diet supplies only very small quantities of calcium, in corn meal and certain vegetables. Taking a calcium supplement to provide 1000 to 1200 mg. per day might be desirable. Ask your physician or nutritionist.

7. If the Aztec diet represents a significant change from your regular eating style, consult your physician and nutritionist before you change over.

The foods that promoted such good health for the Aztecs are, fortunately, widely available today. The biggest differences are in the fruits.

The Aztecs had a wider choice of tropical fruits than we may, but many tropical items—like papaya and guava juices—are often found in health food stores and in some supermarkets, either bottled or as frozen concentrate.

The Aztecs knew their health and energy were tied to the foods they ate. They felt their best when they followed the calendar cycles closely. Life pulsed all around them, with opportunities and changes, birth and growth, learning and love, family and deep bonds. Food was a connection to all these basics of life. They sustained life with food, celebrated with food, and honored their gods with the foods that represented their toil and reverence.

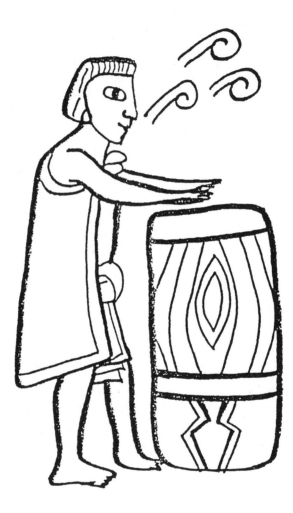

6
Menus for the Days
of the Aztec Calendar

The first day after the five Dead Days they would come. It was the time for renewal, the time for rededication and new beginnings. Those who lived close by would arrive in the first light of morning when the parrots all joined in the mighty endeavor of calling forth the sun. They now would stand quietly, the mother a little teary-eyed as she pulled at the hem of her son's shirt or adjusted the strap of his sandal. The father would be stoic, his pride showing only in the possessive way his hand lay on his son's shoulder.

They would stand at the back of the main pyramid for as long as two or three hours until the priest in charge of apprentices would arrive. Then with little ado they would give their sons to be servants and students to the priests. In the long, thatched abode buildings near the main square the boys would begin hearing and singing the great chants and story-poems repeated again and again until their memory was clear and perfect.

By day the great chants would rise from the temples and platforms on top of the carefully aligned and precisely constructed pyramids. The deep-toned, booming sounds of large hollow logs reverberated through the trees surrounding the pyramid squares. Smaller drums of turtle bodies, large gourds, and curved wooden bowls added variety and musical melodies of their own. Rattles in the shapes of hollow lances, curved horns, and long, decorated arrows added staccato emphasis and sustained excitement to the words of the songs. To the priests fell the strenuous, cosmic work of maintaining the universe in order. They charted and studied the powers of the sun and moon and stars.

By night, it was the quiet voices of the old people in the family that would be heard as they taught about Mother Earth and her gifts to her children. They spoke of the life force in the plants and animals around them.

To the old ones came the task of maintaining the family in order.

Gently, the old hands smoothed the straight, shiny hair of the children seated so close to them. Their soft, old voices talked of opposites and how opposites give meaning to life. They spoke of things the children had experienced and could understand, such as hot and cold, times of work and times of rest, and laughter and tears. They spoke of times of fasting and times of feasting, and the need for each other. And they spoke of times to eat things of the earth, times to eat things of the water, and times to eat things of the air.

Nourished since earliest memory in the rhythm of the calendar, the old ones spoke comfortably of its stories, for the balance and power of the calendar had proved itself again and again.

Day 1

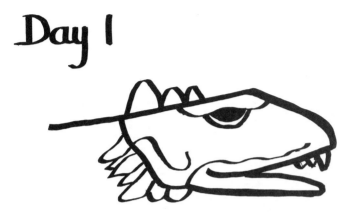

Crocodile

Silver flashes
   Through moving water
Quick, turn,
   Vanish.

Quickness......Power of Fish

DAY 1

CROCODILE

THE QUICKNESS OF THE CROCODILE, a creature of both land and sea and a fierce predator in water, is evident in its ability to catch fish, even though they themselves are quick and elusive in their moves, strands of silver shining in the water.

This quickness comes by eating fish this day.

A number of larger, freshwater lakes near Mexico City provided most of the fish in Aztec times. These lakes had both a rosy- and a white-meat fish 8 to 12 inches long, which the Aztecs caught in nets similar to the often-photographed "butterfly nets." They usually broiled their catch over coals or sautéed them in a light sauce. The fish were prepared whole and not fileted.

A good choice for today would be broiled trout, although a whitefish or haddock filet sautéed in the golden sauce would serve well also. The sauce is mild and brings out the sweetness of the fish.

Symbol	*Food*	*Power*
CROCODILE	FISH	QUICKNESS

Principal Meal
Clear Chives Broth, p. 131
Fish: Broiled trout, whitefish, or haddock or Golden Fish (p. 159)
Tomato and jicama slices, p. 168
Savory Frijoles Refritos, p. 141

Morning
Morning Rain, p. 163
Several pieces of different kinds of citrus fruit: orange, grapefruit,
    tangerine, or tangelo.
Sun Coins (tortillas), p. 170, warmed and topped with honey.

Midmorning
Hot beverage of your choice
Aztec Muffins (p. 163) or whole-wheat English muffins.
Handful (⅓ cup) roasted sunflower seeds, salted or unsalted.

Evening
2–3 Sun Coins (tortillas), p. 170
Vegetable Plate of steamed carrots, parsnips, and potatoes.

CROCODILE—FISH

HEALTHY INGREDIENTS AND COMBINATIONS

There are two low-calorie protein sources for this day: the beans/tortillas and the fish. The fish suggested in the recipe section, trout, whitefish, or haddock, have only about 3 grams of fat per ounce. Fish has an added advantage the fact that the fats are omega-3 fatty acids, which are polyunsaturated fats. Fish are also a good source of certain vitamins, especially thiamine and niacin.

The evening steamed vegetable platter is high in fiber, low in fat, and moderate in protein. The parsnips and potatoes provide potassium, and the carrots are an excellent source of beta carotene.

The other fruits and vegetables provide vitamins, minerals, fiber, and carbohydrates. The muffins and tortillas also provide nutritious carbohydrates.

Day 2

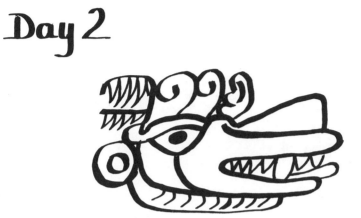

Wind

Bow down the trees,
Move the clouds,
Tear them open,
Give rain to the crops.

Strength.....Power of
Vegetables

DAY 2

WIND

Strong winds accompany the heavy thundershowers that bring the needed rain for the crops. The strength that brings the clouds and rain is given to the crops, which can be dried to give life all winter. Baked in its own husks in a tamale, ground corn is one of the prime foods that gives this strength.

Corn was an important symbol of fertility for the Aztecs. The tall top flower waits for the wind to shake pollen onto the waiting ears below. If watered deeply, the plant could withstand intense sun and heat and still yield a crop. It was the plant of the sun god, with its golden kernels that could be ground and shaped into tortillas, round and golden like the sun —Sun Coins.

Symbol	*Food*	*Power*
WIND	SWEET TAMALES	STRENGTH

Principal Meal
   Painted Squash Stew, p. 142
   Sweet Little Tamales, p. 156
   Peanut brittle

Morning
   Morning Rain, p. 163
   Meal: Several pieces of assorted sweet fruits—apples, pears, bananas
   3–4 Sun Coins (p. 170), warmed, topped with honey.

Midmorning
   Hot chocolate
   Whole-wheat rolls
   Handful (⅓ cup) pumpkin seeds

Evening
   Sun Coin stack (p. 170)
   Vegetable Plate of sliced tomatoes, cucumbers, and cauliflower

WIND—SWEET TAMALES
HEALTHY INGREDIENTS AND COMBINATIONS

The Painted Squash Stew is rich in vitamins and protein. The bell pepper provides vitamin C, and the squash and carrots are rich in vitamin A in the form of beta carotene. The squash also provides some protein while being low in fat. The beans in the stew add proteins and carbohydrates.

The tamales are rich in B vitamins and carbohydrates.

The fruits and vegetables suggested for breakfast, snacks, and evening meal are also good sources of vitamins and fiber, and the accompanying rolls and tortillas have vitamins, fiber, and carbohydrates.

Day 3

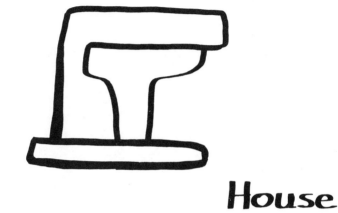

House

Sound the drum,
Play the flute
Adorn your door with flowers
And your heart with song

Love of home .... Power of
this feast

DAY 3

HOUSE

HOME WAS IMPORTANT to the Aztecs, and family bonds and obligations were treated with respect. Marriage was so important in their society that adultery was punished by execution. This feast day commemorated family bonds. It was a holiday celebrated with lavish amounts of food and family visits.

Turkey was one of the favorite feast foods of the Aztecs, and its domestication by the Mayas before the time of Christ made it a reliable food source. Turkeys were cooked whole on a spit over coals, something like rotisserie cooking today, or roasted in an outdoor oven. Preparation often depended on the weather, just as our barbecues today are seasonal. Turkeys were also cut up and prepared in various sauces, the most famous being *mole* (MOE-leh), a chocolate-based sauce. This is an unusual, slightly spicy dish. The chocolate is not presweetened, giving this dish a unique flavor. It is the main dish for today.

Symbol	*Food*	*Power*
HOUSE	TURKEY (feast)	LOVE OF HOME

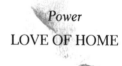

Principal Meal
  Vegetable Soup, p. 132
  Tomato and jicama slices
  Turkey mole, p. 148

  Corn Bread (p. 165), baked thin and drizzled with honey
                              or
  Fresh or frozen ears of corn

  Nahua Squash, p. 149
  Sweet Pockets, p. 166

Morning
  Morning Rain, p. 163
  Honey Rolls (p. 164) or purchased sweet rolls
  Sweet and juicy fruits, especially summer items of cantaloupe and

honeydew melon; in winter, canned or frozen peaches or melon balls.

Midmorning
Tropical juices: papaya, guava, pineapple

Evening
Turkey Tortilla Rolls, p. 167
Tomato, Jicama, and Chive Marinade, p. 168

HOME—TURKEY

HEALTHY INGREDIENTS AND COMBINATIONS

The vegetable soup at the beginning of the meal followed by the tomato and jicama slices provide vitamin A and vitamin C in easily digested form.

The turkey is high in complete protein. It is a good source of B vitamins, especially when cooked in a sauce like the mole, since the sauce retains the natural juices containing the water-soluble B vitamins. Turkey is also a good source of organic iron, which is readily used by the body.

The corn bread, corn, and squash are good sources of carbohydrates and fiber.

Because this is a feast day, there is an emphasis on sweet fruits, especially melons, that are rich in vitamins A and C and also potassium.

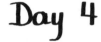

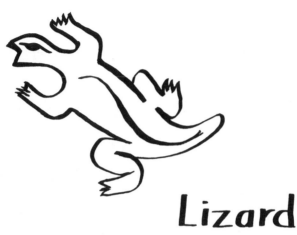

Lizard

Running in the sun,
 Resting in the shade,
Living through drought
 By hiding in the earth.

Endurance ..... Power of
             Vegetables-underground

∧∧∧∧∧∧∧∧∧∧∧∧∧∧∧∧∧∧∧∧∧∧

DAY 4

LIZARD

WHEN THE FIERCE midday sun drives everything to seek the shelter of some shady spot, the lizard digs into the cool sand. He emerges as brightly colored as he entered, even after periods of no rain, seemingly able to survive indefinitely. From vegetables grown underground where the lizard hides comes the power to endure.

Like all crops that are toiled over, vegetables give back strength and vigor. Prepared simply, either raw (if suitable for the particular vegetable), or boiled until tender, vegetables were served with minimum cooking time and maximum eye appeal. Ever aware of color, the Aztec cook's selection was based on appearance as well as taste.

The cazuela (cass-WELL-ah) for today could easily be prepared in a crock pot on low heat.

Symbol	*Food*	*Power*
LIZARD	VEGETABLES GROWN UNDERGROUND	ENDURANCE

Principal Meal
 Cazuela of Cassava or Sweet Potatoes, p. 149
 Nopal fig (Prickly pear fruit, or substitute pineapple rings)
 Sweet Rolled Tortillas, p. 166

Morning
 Morning Rain, p. 163
 Citrus fruits such as oranges or grapefruit
 Tortillas, if desired

Midmorning
 Beverage
 Aztec Muffins (p. 163) or whole-wheat English muffins
 Handful about (½ cup total) salted peanuts, raisins, and shredded
  coconut, mixed

Evening
   Clear Onion Broth, p. 131
   Rolls
   Vegetable Plate with carrot sticks and jicama slices

LIZARD—VEGETABLES

HEALTHY INGREDIENTS AND COMBINATIONS

Today's main dish, the cazuela, uses the deep-yellow or orange vegetables that are rich in vitamin A and vitamin B. The 1988 surgeon general's *Report on Nutrition and Health* cites studies that show that these vitamins may help to prevent cancer of the larynx, esophagus, and lungs.

The citrus fruits of the morning meal contain vitamin C, and the tortillas and muffins provide carbohydrates and vitamin B.

Today's foods provide generous amounts of carbohydrates, fats, vitamins, and minerals. The foods of the main meal of the day are not devoid of protein, but do not contain the full recommended amount of approximately 50 grams per day. Be sure to eat the peanuts suggested in the midmorning snack, if not at that time, then at some other time, since they will provide the additional protein. (Peanuts contain 7 grams of protein per ounce.)

Day 5

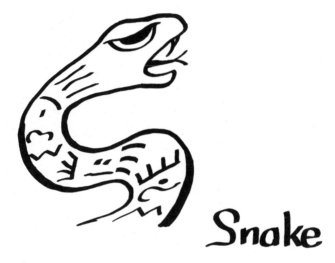

Snake

Touching Mother Earth
With all your body
Yet ascending to the sun
On mystic plumes.

Meditation ..... Power of Eggs

DAY 5

SNAKE

ONE OF THE CENTRAL FIGURES of Aztec worship was Quetzalcoatl (kehtz-all-COH-ah-tl), the Feathered Serpent. His head and open, fanged mouth, carefully carved in limestone, adorn many of the Aztec monuments near Mexico City. Also, if you look at the Aztec calendar (page 7), the other rim represents two snakes, their tails at the top and their mouths at the bottom, with a human face inside each mouth, one white and one black. The squares around the rim are stylized representations of scales.

Snakes were a sign of power and renewal, for they emerge glistening and vibrant after shedding their skins. Also, snakes often eat eggs, another symbol of renewal. This day has two renewal symbols, the snake and the egg, for eating eggs this day provides access to spiritual powers.

As messengers to the gods, snakes were thought to aid prayer and meditation. The Aztecs made meditation a part of their religious life, and they felt spiritually uplifted and renewed by it.

The Aztecs ate turkey eggs, which are very similar to the hen eggs we eat today. Eggs were usually served with another food, and the Feathered Serpent Beans would be a typical dish in which the eggs are served on top of the beans, then covered with a chili sauce.

Symbol	*Food*	*Power*
SNAKE	EGGS	MEDITATION

Principal Meal
Parsley Broth, p. 133
Feathered Serpent Beans, p. 150
Squash Boats, p. 151
Sweet Rolled Tortillas, p. 166

Morning
Morning Rain, p. 163
Sweet fruits, such as banana, apple, cherries
Aztec Omelette, p. 165

Midmorning
   Juice
   Handful (⅓ cup) pumpkin seeds

Evening
   Corn Soup, p. 165
   Tomato Tostada, p. 167

SNAKE—EGGS

HEALTHY INGREDIENTS AND COMBINATIONS

The main meal today features the classic, simple Aztec foods that constituted such a healthy diet. The beans and tortillas combine to form a complete protein, in which all twenty-two amino acids are present for nutritional use. Eggs provide additional complete protein, which is easily digested and absorbed.

The beans and tortillas also provide carbohydrates and vitamin B. The other fruits and vegetables suggested for the day offer vitamin A and vitamin C and fiber.

The Corn Soup and Tomato Tostada of the evening are especially rich in vitamin A, vitamin C, and potassium, and provide a small amount of calcium as well.

Day 6

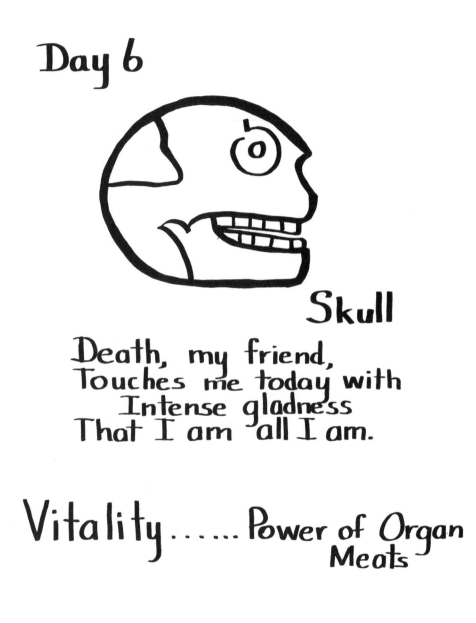

Skull

Death, my friend,
Touches me today with
    Intense gladness
That I am all I am.

Vitality......Power of Organ
            Meats

DAY 6

SKULL

To THE AZTECS, death was the ever-present, necessary opposite of life. Since life was so treasured, a human life was the ultimate and best sacrifice possible. An honorable death, especially in battle or as a sacrifice, became the door to life with the gods. Their awareness of death as "the other half of life" is graphically and dramatically shown in certain Tlatilco sculptures that portrayed seated figures divided down the midline of the body with normal body structure and skin on one side and a skeleton and skull on the other.

The Aztecs were well versed in anatomy and aware of the functions of the vital organs. The day of Skull was a day of awareness of life and the vital organs that sustained it. By partaking of organ meats, such as heart or liver, they increased their own vitality.

Bittersweets reflect the awareness of life's opposites by mixing the slightly acrid taste of chicken liver with the sweetness of pineapple. The combination creates a piquant and pleasant dish.

Symbol	*Food*	*Power*
SKULL	ORGAN MEATS	VITALITY

Principal Meal
    Vegetable Soup, p. 132
    Bittersweets (Chicken livers), p. 152,
        served on
    Corn Bread, p. 165
    Savory Frijoles Refritos, p. 141

Morning
    Morning Rain, p. 163
    Vine fruits, like melon and grapes
    Sun Coins, topped with honey

Midmorning
    Hot chocolate
    Amaranth rolls

Evening
   Tortilla Soup, p. 137
   Vegetable Plate p. 164
   Aztec Muffins (p. 163) or whole-wheat English muffins

SKULL—ORGAN MEATS

HEALTHY INGREDIENTS AND COMBINATIONS

The Vegetable Soup at the beginning of the main meal provides vitamin A and vitamin C. The Tortilla Soup at the end of the day also provides those same vitamins, along with carbohydrates.

The chicken-liver dish in the main meal is high in protein and also contains vitamin A, vitamin C, riboflavin, niacin, and vitamins B_6 and B_{12}. It also is a rich source of organic iron that is easily absorbed by the body.

The Corn Bread and tortillas and rolls provide carbohydrates and B vitamins plus calcium.

The fresh fruits and vegetables suggested for the day provide carbohydrates, vitamins, and fiber.

Day 7

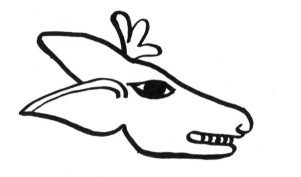

Deer

Moving in shadows
Watching, listening
Darting on arrow feet
Watching, listening.

Alertness.....Power of Deer

DAY 7

DEER

HUNTING WAS AN ADMIRED SKILL among the Aztecs because silent movement in the jungle underbrush is difficult. Trees and bushes can create a wall that has openings large enough to admit the deer but not the hunter. Fleetness and caution are the powers of this day that help the deer survive. The Aztecs admired them for their alertness.

The deer that live in the tropic and subtropic regions of Mexico are a little smaller than many of the species of our country. They were hunted with bow and arrow as a source of food. The meat was often cut into thin strips and broiled over coals, or simmered in a sauce, then wrapped in a tortilla to be served. *Mazatl* is the Aztec word for deer, and Mazatles are small bits of meat, such as tenderloin tips or kebob squares, cut thin, simmered in a spicy sauce, and served in a rolled, soft tortilla.

Deer meat also lends itself to drying or smoking for preservation, and after drying it was prepared in a dish that simmered the meat to reconstitute it. Then it was fixed as a *tamal*, an Aztec word describing spiced meat in a blanket of ground corn meal that was wrapped in corn husks so it could easily be roasted by being placed in a bed of coals.

For ease of preparation today, the basic ingredients can easily be prepared in a baking dish (see Tamale Casserole, p. 153) instead of corn husks. The corn husks on tamales were not a necessary part of the recipe, only a handy, inexpensive, biodegradable cooking container.

Symbol	*Food*	*Power*
DEER	DEER, WILD GAME (Sliced or Ground Meat)	ALERTNESS

Principal Meal
Chive Broth, p. 131
Mazatles, p. 158
   or
Tamale Casserole, p. 153

Baked Sweet Potatoes
Amaranth-Nopal Fritters, p. 168

Morning
    Morning Rain, p. 163
    Citrus fruits: orange, tangerines
    Sun Coins topped with honey

Midmorning
    Juice
    Aztec Muffins, p. 163, or purchased whole-wheat English muffins
    Handful (⅓ cup) sunflower seeds, raisins, and peanuts, mixed

Evening
    Vegetable Plate, p. 164
    Sweet Pockets, p. 166

DEER—MAZATLES

HEALTHY INGREDIENTS AND COMBINATIONS

The Mazatles suggested for today were prepared with venison in Aztec times. Deer provides an animal-source protein, and the meat of the deer is typically much leaner than the beef we are accustomed to eating. Deer meat does not have the fat marbling, but the protein contributions of the two meats are roughly equal, and lean pieces of beef represent an appropriate substitution. The meat provides niacin, vitamins B_6 and B_{12}, and iron.

The sweet potatoes add vitamin A and B vitamins as well as complex carbohydrates and fiber.

The citrus fruits of the morning provide vitamin C and some natural fiber.

The vegetables recommended for the evening are important additions for the day, since they provide fiber and many additional vitamins.

Day 8

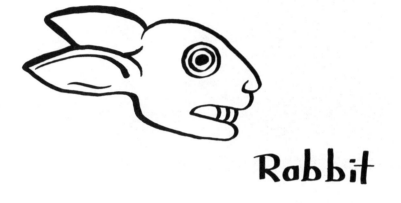

Rabbit

As fast as the
South Wind,
Only the eagle
Can catch you as you run.

Speed .... Power of Rabbit

DAY 8

RABBIT

THE AZTECS DID NOT HAVE any sort of animal transportation, such as horses, so runners working in relays formed an important part of the emperor's information network. Foot races of various kinds were common games for children, and a young man from a poor family who cultivated a natural running skill could win a place on a relay squad in the emperor's guard, improving his economic and social status. Speed was a desirable power, one that could be acquired in eating rabbit meat.

Rabbits were hunted with snares and also with an *atl-atl*, a curved board with a groove down the center that could hold a dart (in this case) or a spear. It was swung through the air, and the dart was released at just the right instant. It significantly increased the speed and distance of the projectile compared to throwing the dart or spear by hand.

You could use either rabbit or chicken in the main dish for today. The taste of the two meats is similar, as is their texture, and if you do not care for rabbit, chicken is a good, if not authentic, substitute. The Aztecs used chili in many of their dishes, but not everyone ate the very hottest chili all the time. In fact, their personal culinary tastes varied as much as ours do. Use your own taste to decide how much spice you would like, for there is no set piquancy that would make this dish any more or less authentic.

Symbol	*Food*	*Power*
RABBIT	RABBIT (Chicken)	SPEED

Principal Meal
Corn Soup, p. 134
Spicy Rabbit or Chicken, p. 154
Mixed Vegetables with Tomato Salsa, p. 168
Sun Coins, p. 170

Morning
Morning Rain, p. 163
Fruit Compote, p. 170
Whole-wheat rolls

Midmorning
  Hot beverage
  Aztec Muffins, p. 163, or whole-wheat English muffins
  Handful (⅓ cup) pumpkin seeds

Evening
  Vegetable Tamale Pie, p. 145
  Tomato and jicama slices

RABBIT—RABBIT OR CHICKEN

HEALTHY INGREDIENTS AND COMBINATIONS

On Day Rabbit you may use either rabbit or chicken, since both are light meats with less fat than beef, pork, or lamb. They also have similar tastes and textures. Either one is a complete protein source, with vitamin B in the juices. The baked recipe for this day is a low-fat way to prepare either meat, since no oils are used in the cooking. Rabbit in the store comes skinned. If using chicken, reduce the fat content further by skinning the meat before dredging it in the spices.

The Fruit Compote blends several kinds of fruits together, providing vitamin A and vitamin C. The exact quantity of these vitamins varies, depending on the fruits selected.

The Vegetable Tamale Pie and the Mixed Vegetables in a slightly spicy sauce all provide carbohydrates, vitamins A and C, and fiber.

Day 9

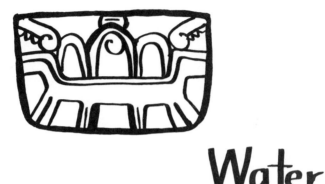

Water

Rippling, moving, calling.
Glistening. Shining,
The promise of freshness
Held in splashing song.

Cleanliness.....Power of Water

DAY 9

WATER

THE YUCCA PLANT grows naturally from the Southwestern United States desert down to Panama. If you pull up the plant and dry the roots you can make an excellent soap and shampoo. To make the soap you peel back the outer layer of the root, place the whole root in a fairly large container of water, then beat the water vigorously with your hand. In a few moments you will have a sudsy solution ready to use.

On any given workday you would have seen Aztec women flocking to lake or stream banks and kneeling patiently on rocks by the water and scrubbing the family's clothes, then laying them on nearby rocks to dry. They were able to get their white clothes brilliantly white by leaving the yucca lather on the cloth and letting it bleach in the sun for several hours before they were rinsed. Natural hot springs were important ritual bathing spots, and regular streams and lakes were used daily by the Aztecs for bathing, even in cool weather. They prized cleanliness and appreciated the spiritual force of water for its cleansing power.

Day Water was a day for cleansing. Only one meal was eaten, although water was taken liberally throughout the day. This was a holiday for the Aztecs. They neither worked in the fields nor held market. Religious ceremonies were held at various temples.

In our American culture we have a strong pioneer heritage and traditions based in country living with emphasis on hearty nutrition and the ideal of three meals a day. It is not our tradition to rest or cleanse the system. The Aztecs found that good nutrition does not necessarily mean three solid meals a day. They had excellent results with this partial fast once during the twenty days.

Those people with a medical condition, such as diabetes, in which fasting would be harmful, or who need to take medication accompanied by food, should consult their physician before beginning even this partial fast.

Fish, which live in water, are the meal for today. Huachinango (wah-chee-NAN-go)—red snapper—or catfish filets would be a good choice for today. The Huachinango recipe makes a sauce that is suitable for filets of most mild-flavored fish.

Symbol	Food	Power
WATER	FISH	CLEANLINESS

Holiday; a fast day; water cleansing
Only one meal taken in the late afternoon
Water is taken freely throughout the day, at least 8 oz. every three
  hours.

Late Afternoon
  Fish: Huachinango, p. 141
  Aztec Beans, p. 142
  Sun Coins, p. 170

WATER—FISH

HEALTHY INGREDIENTS AND COMBINATIONS

The intent of this day was a partial fast, in which generous amounts of
water were taken, about one 8-oz. glass every three hours.

The one meal of the day provides protein and B vitamins in the fish,
and carbohydrates and additional protein in the beans. The beans combine with the tortillas (Sun Coins) to provide a complete protein as well
as niacin, B vitamins, and fiber.

Day 10

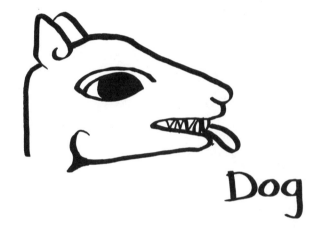

Dog

In spasms of barking
You try to speak,
    But you forgot the words
And howl in sadness.

Loyalty........ Power of Lamb

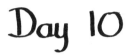

DAY 10

DOG

MOST OF US find the Aztec habit of eating dog thoroughly unappetizing, but this aversion is based for the most part on cultural bias. It is not unusual for one culture to find the practices of another quite distasteful. To the Hindu our practice of raising cattle to eat is barbaric, and several Mid-Eastern religions forbid the eating of pork, the principal ingredient of that American staple, the hot dog. What is unusual about the Aztecs eating dog is that very few carnivores are common sources of food in any culture, ancient or modern. With the exception of carnivorous fish, and pigs, which are omnivores, most cultures do not make carnivorous predators a regular part of their diet. But the Aztecs did raise dogs, appreciated their trait of loyalty, and did eat them.

The dogs they raised for food were small, something like a modern Chihuahua. Often the thighs and back were the main pieces used. They were cut into small pieces and prepared in a stew.

The Aztecs did not have lamb, but it is suggested here as an acceptable substitution for our Day Dog meal. In the Olla (OH-yah) Lamb recipe (p. 143) one ingredient listed is jicama (HEE-cah-mah), a Mexican vegetable that is grown underground. With the increasing popularity of Mexican foods, jicama is finding a wider and wider market, and you should find it in the vegetable section of the grocery store. It is shaped like a large light-brown beet. The light-brown outer layer is peeled or cut off. The inside of the plant is white and sweet and crisp. It can be cut into thin bite-sized slices and served raw. It can also be cooked and has the delightful quality of staying rather crisp even when cooked. If not available in your area, russet or small red potatoes are just as delicious in this recipe.

Symbol	*Food*	*Power*
DOG	LAMB	LOYALTY

Principal Meal
  Olla Lamb, p. 143
  Corn Bread, p. 165
  Tomato and jicama slices

Morning
　　Morning Rain, p. 163
　　Sweet fruits: banana and pear
　　Warm tortillas with honey and cinnamon

Midmorning
　　Hot chocolate or other beverage
　　Sweet rolls

Evening
　　Sweet Rolled Tortillas, p. 166
　　Vegetable Plate, p. 164

DOG—LAMB

HEALTHY INGREDIENTS AND COMBINATIONS

Lamb is a reasonable substitution for dog this day, since lamb provides an animal source of complete protein and lends itself to the stew kind of dish that is typical of the day. The lamb provides organic iron and niacin and vitamin B_{12}.

The fruits provide carbohydrates, vitamin C, and potassium.

The tortillas, corn bread, and rolls add additional carbohydrates and a small amount of calcium.

The vegetables in the Olla Lamb dish are a good source of vitamins, carbohydrates, and fiber, as are the vegetables in the evening Vegetable Plate.

Day 11

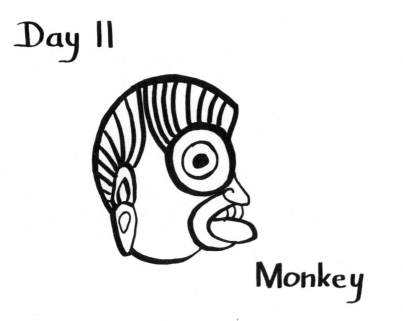

Monkey

The fruit I must climb for
You reach with ease,
Swinging, gliding, never dropping
Your baby from your hairy arms.

Agility........Power of Fruits

∿∿∿∿∿∿∿∿∿∿∿∿∿∿∿

DAY 11

MONKEY

THE AZTEC CAPITAL OF TENOCHTITLÁN was on a plateau at an elevation of about 8,000 feet. Yet the Aztecs were not isolated from the surrounding lands. The tropical lowlands, a two-day journey by foot from the capital, played an important role in Aztec life. Their produce and animals are well represented in Aztec symbols.

One of the animals often depicted are the monkeys that live in the lowlands. These small treetop dwellers live on fruit and are admired for their agility. The Aztecs enhanced this power in themselves by eating fruit on this day.

The Fruit Skewers recipe is typical of many of the tropical dishes you might still find in Mexico today. It had many seasonal variations, but the basic preparation was the same. Several different fruits were cut into cubes that were easy to handle and thread on a wooden skewer. These were coated with a honey-based sauce that was sticky enough to adhere to the fruit while it was braised over coals.

Symbol	*Food*	*Power*
MONKEY	FRUITS	AGILITY

Principal Meal
  Fruit Skewers, p. 147
  Palm Treat Tortillas, p. 169

Morning
  Morning Rain, p. 163
  Summer fruits: cherries, apricot, peach (frozen or canned if not in season)
  Honey Rolls, p. 164

Midmorning
  Herbal tea
  Warm Sun Coins with honey and cinnamon
  Handful (⅓ cup) peanuts and dried banana chips

Evening
   Fruit Compote, p. 170
   Rolls

MONKEY—FRUITS

HEALTHY INGREDIENTS AND COMBINATIONS

Fruits are naturally high in sugar, providing energy in the form of carbohydrate. Fruits are low in protein, however, meaning that less than 5 percent of their calories are provided by proteins. The fruits of the main meal suggested for today are especially rich in vitamins.

The bananas are high in potassium and magnesium and also contain B vitamins. The mangoes are especially high in vitamin A in the form of betacarotene, which is the form the American Cancer Society says may afford some protection against cancers induced by chemicals. Papayas are similarly colored and rich in vitamin A and are also rich in potassium. The pineapple is a good source of vitamin C.

Eating fruit and grain products like tortillas and rolls make this a high-carbohydrate day. If you are like most people who do this for one day, you will feel light and energetic.

As I go through the rotation of the Aztec calendar I look forward to this day because I really enjoy the sweet Fruit Skewers in the main meal. I can see how the Aztecs felt agile on this day, since I felt the lift of the fruit sugars and the light digestive load.

Day 12

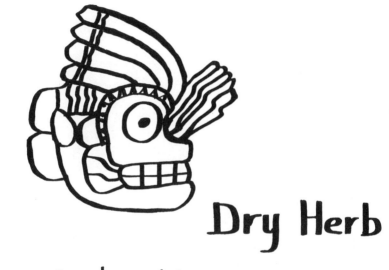

Dry Herb

Now in trembling pain
Yet I feel healing begin;
Herbs cover the wound,
My flesh will close again.

Healing ......Power of Herbs

DAY 12

DRY HERB

AZTEC PHYSICIANS were very well versed in the medicinal effects of many of the plants and herbs of the empire. With the area's great variety of climate and terrain, they came to know a great assortment of medicinal plants. They used tranquilizers for trauma and loss, and purgatives for suspected "bad spirits." Healing herb pastes were applied directly to skin for injuries. They were also versed on various hallucinogens (magic mushrooms), although these did not create a "drug" problem for the Aztecs since mind-altering plants were strictly associated with religious rites, mostly for the males, and were not used regularly.

The Aztec traditions of using various herbs and plants for healing are kept alive even today through *curanderas* or *curanderos* (coo-ran-DER-ohs). These are, literally, village healers who have a wide stock of herbal concoctions that are often quite effective in treating various maladies. Researchers today are working diligently to record as much of these verbal traditions as possible, since some of our medicines today are derived from tropical plants used by these folk healers. Their belief in the efficacy of the herbs was an additional factor in the success of their remedies. With the herbs used in today's meal, the Aztecs sought healing for sadness as much as for any physical discomfort.

The Butternut Soup with Herbs that is the main dish for today uses three sweet herbs for flavor. The butternut squash as the base of the soup has a rich flavor of its own, which is greatly enhanced by the herbs. Don't be surprised if you find yourself wanting more than one bowl— and since it is low-calorie, help yourself!

Symbol	*Food*	*Power*
DRY HERB	VEGETABLE/HERB SOUPS, STEWS	HEALING

Principal Meal
Butternut Soup with Herbs, p. 135
Aztec Beans, p. 142
Sun Coins, p. 170
Mixed Nuts

Morning
   Morning Rain, p. 163
   Citrus fruits: grapefruit, orange, tangerine
   Sun Coins with honey, p. 170

Midmorning
   Hot beverage
   Aztec Muffins, p. 163, or whole-wheat English muffins
   Handful (⅓ cup) pumpkin seeds

Evening
   Vegetable Plate, p. 164
   Whole-wheat rolls

DRY HERB—VEGETABLE HERB

HEALTHY INGREDIENTS AND COMBINATIONS

The soup that is today's main dish has squash as the principal ingredient. This is one of the orange-yellow vegetables that is high in the carotenoids that the body converts to Vitamin A and that the American Cancer Society suggests as an important nutrient for the prevention of cancers of the respiratory system. Combined with the tortillas and the nuts served with the main meal, there is complete protein provided, along with vitamin B, Iron, and phosphorous. Pumpkin seeds, sprinkled generously on the evening Vegetable Plate, will also provide some iron, phosphorous, and vitamin E.

The citrus fruits suggested for the morning meal are high in vitamin C and provide moderate amounts of fiber. The tortillas and rolls offer carbohydrates and complete the proteins in the vegetables. The nuts are high in unsaturated fats and add protein and vitamin B to the day's foods.

Day 13

From water where fish hide
And from dark, wet earth
The reed rises, strong and straight
To become the musical flute.

Music .... Power of Fish

DAY 13

REED/CANE

FLUTES AND DRUMS were the main Aztec musical instruments and accompanied singing. We know this from mural scenes which show ceremonies of various sorts in which drummers, flutists, and singers are obviously providing accompaniment. We don't have any of the music in its original form. However, musicologists feel that some of the folk music forms still heard in Mexico today may have some of the ancient rhythms and melodies. They feel this is true because of the great musical diversity of the different regions of Mexico. We do know that music was important to the Aztecs, who felt this power was acquired by eating fish this day, for fish live among the reeds from which flutes were made.

On this day, as on Day 1 (Crocodile), a small whole fish such as trout would be the most authentic choice, but a light-meated filet of perch or cod would do just as well. A special recipe that is more typical of the coastal region is included for today, using a special spiced lemon-honey-butter sauce.

Symbol	*Food*	*Power*
REED/CANE	FISH	MUSIC

Principal Meal
Clear Chives Broth, p. 131
Golden Fish, p. 159
Corn Bread, p. 165

Morning
Morning Rain, p. 163
Sweet fruits: apple, pear, banana
Sun Coins, p. 170

Midmorning
Fruit juices
Honey Rolls, p. 164
Shredded coconut, peanuts, and raisins (mixed—total about ½ cup)

Evening
  Deep Dish Corn, p. 152
  Savory Frijoles Refritos, p. 141
  Rolls

REED/CANE—FISH

HEALTHY INGREDIENTS AND COMBINATIONS

The Vegetable Soup that begins the main meal of the day provides vitamin A, vitamin C, and potassium. The corn meal in the Corn Bread has carbohydrates, vitamin B, and calcium. The fish is a complete protein source and also provides B vitamins, iodine, selenium, phosphorus, iron, and calcium. The fish dish also contains polyunsaturated oils from its ingredients and the natural fish oils.

The Frijoles Refritos and the corn casserole have an abundance of carbohydrates and polyunsaturated oils as well as additional vitamin A and B vitamins.

The fruits of the day provide fiber, vitamins, and additional carbohydrates in the form of fructose, which is very easy to assimilate.

Day 14

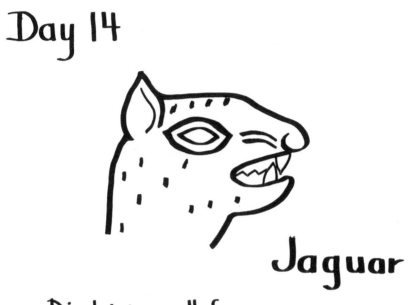

Jaguar

Disdaining all fear,
   Walking in total grace
With terrible teeth, terrible claws
   And terrible beauty.

Grace ...... Power of this Feast

DAY 14

JAGUAR

THE JAGUAR was an important god to the Aztecs. He represented grace, power, and beauty. To liken someone to a jaguar was a great compliment, and boys born on Day Jaguar were likely to receive a name connected to the animal or one of its attributes. Jaguar pelts were prized and were worn by Aztec nobility as a symbol of high rank. Warriors and athletes were also entitled to wear them as rewards for valor or success.

Day Jaguar was a feast day with emphasis on athletic events. The feast of this day is connected to the power of being lithe and graceful.

Since turkey is a feast food, it is used once again on this feast day. The Aztecs slow-roasted it, wrapped in banana leaves. To simulate this method practically, I used two paper sacks like those typically found at the grocery store. The turkey is prepared whole with several spices rubbed on the skin. Then it is placed inside the sacks and roasted at a low temperature for a long time. Meat cooked in this fashion is unusually tender.

Symbol	*Food*	*Power*
JAGUAR	TURKEY (feast)	GRACE

Principal Meal
  Vegetable Soup, p. 132
  Slow Roast Turkey, p. 157

  Thin Corn Bread, p. 165
     or
  Roasted ears of corn

  Aztec Beans, p. 142
  Sweet Pockets, p. 166

Morning
  Morning Rain, p. 163
  Honey Rolls, p. 164
  Fruit basket, special fruit items: apricot, peach, pear, grapes

Midmorning
Tropical juices: papaya, guava, pineapple
Nuts (your favorite)

Evening
Nahua Squash, p. 149
Pyramids, p. 144

JAGUAR—TURKEY

HEALTHY INGREDIENTS AND COMBINATIONS

This is a feast day with an emphasis on abundance. The Vegetable Soup that begins the main meal provides vitamins A and C and iron and potassium from the green beans, and vitamin A in the form of betacarotenes from the carrots.

The turkey, especially in this slow-roast recipe, provides riboflavin, vitamins B_6 and B_{12}, and niacin. In addition, it is a good source of organic iron, zinc, and magnesium.

The corn or Corn Bread provide carbohydrates, B vitamins, and a small amount of polyunsaturated fats. The beans and pumpkin dessert yield carbohydrates and additional vitamin A, as do the squash and beans from the evening meal.

The tropical juices are rich in carotene and fructose, and the morning fruits provide additional vitamins C and A and carbohydrate in the form of fructose.

Day 15

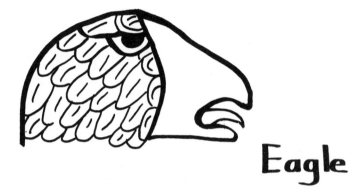

Eagle

My prayers
Are in your feathers
And whisper
When you circle the sky

Spirituality ...... Power of Meat

DAY 15

EAGLE

THE EAGLE was an important symbol to the Aztecs, who believed he could soar to the very center of the heavens if he chose.

The eagle played a major part in the Aztecs' choice of where to establish their capital. According to the legend, as the Aztecs traveled from Aztlan, their home in the north, their leader received a vision. He was told he must travel until he came to a place where he would see an eagle with a snake in its beak sitting on a cactus. That would be the sign that they had reached their new home. At Tenochtitlán that scene occurred, just as foretold, and so it became the birthplace of the Aztec nation.

That legend is portrayed on the Mexican flag today. The colors of the flag are red, white, and green in three broad vertical stripes. In the center stripe, which is white, is the legendary eagle.

By soaring to the center of the sky, the eagle could meet the spirits of the gods. This powerful religious goal for the Aztecs inspired them to thoughts of deity and spiritual worthiness. The power of this day, spirituality, was obtained by eating those things the eagle ate, such as snake and rabbit.

In the menu for today, a substitution of ground meat is made in the dish called Soaring Wings, which is typical of the carefully prepared dishes of a special day like Eagle. Soaring Wings combines the power of the frijol, cultivated in the earth, with the power of the sun in the Sun Coins or tortillas.

Symbol	Food	Power
EAGLE	SNAKE, RABBIT (Substitute: ground meat)	SPIRITUALITY

Principal Meal
Parsley Broth, p. 133
Soaring Wings, p. 155
Fresh jicama slices

Morning
  Morning Rain, p. 163
  Grapes
  Rolls

Midmorning
  Juice
  Handful (⅓ cup) peanuts, shredded coconut

Evening
  Savory Frijoles Refritos, p. 141
  Sun Coins

EAGLE—GROUND MEAT
HEALTHY INGREDIENTS AND COMBINATIONS

It is appropriate to substitute ground meat for the snake the Aztecs might
have eaten. The snake is an animal source of protein, as is the ground
beef suggested in the main recipe for today of Soaring Wings, and since
their recipe uses meat that has been chopped very small, the ground
meat is the best choice.

The Vegetable Soup that begins the main meal of the day is a good
source of vitamins, especially vitamins A and C.

The Soaring Wings recipe combines ground meat, tortillas, pinto
beans, and cream cheese in a tomato sauce. This provides a rich amount
of complete protein, organic iron, B vitamins, and vitamin C. It also
provides carbohydrates and fat.

Additional protein is provided in the beans and tortillas of the evening
meal, as are carbohydrates and vitamin A.

Day 16

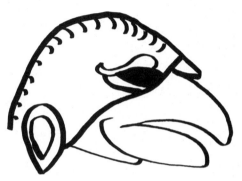

Vulture

You feast on death's leavings,
Taking life from death;
So in my heart,
Hope lives after sorrow.

Hope ...... Power of Stewed
Meats

DAY 16

VULTURE

THE VULTURE does not soar high like the eagle, and on the ground he lumbers and hops in an ungainly way, his bald head bobbing jerkily. But aloft he will ride the air currents in wide, graceful loops for many hours, looking, waiting, wings outstretched, willing to take what is left after the rapacious eagle and proud jaguar have eaten their fill. He perseveres, like hope, even when things seem bleak. The food for this day is properly a stew, pieces of whatever you can find.

Caldo Bueno (KAHL-doe BWEH-no), the main recipe for today, is a kind of stew. This hearty and satisfying dish is usually made with a fair amount of chili, either canned or powdered, but you can vary that to suit your taste.

Symbol	Food	Power
VULTURE	CALDO BUENO	HOPE

Principal Meal
    Caldo Bueno, p. 160
    Corn Bread, p. 165
    Sweet Pockets, p. 166

Morning
    Morning Rain, p. 163
    Citrus fruits: grapefruit, orange
    Aztec Muffins, p. 163, or whole-wheat English muffins

Midmorning
    Hot beverage
    Sun Coins with honey
    Mixed peanuts, banana chips, sunflower seeds (about ½ cup)

Evening
    Tortilla Soup, p. 137
    Vegetable Tamale Pie, p. 145

VULTURE—STEW

HEALTHY INGREDIENTS AND COMBINATIONS

The Caldo Bueno stew that is the main meal for today offers a cornucopia of nutrients. The ground meat has animal-source iron and complete protein, which increases the protein quality of the squash and corn. The tomatoes are rich in vitamin A and vitamin C, and the potatoes provide carbohydrates and potassium.

The citrus fruits of the morning provide vitamin C and fiber and carbohydrates in the form of natural fructose.

The Tortilla Soup has vitamin C, B vitamins, and vitamin A, and also provides a small amount of calcium.

Day 17

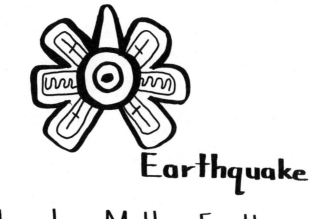

Earthquake

In her sleep Mother Earth
Forgets to cradle her children
And dreams.....and sighs....
And moves.

Sensitivity........Power of Vegetables

‸‸‸‸‸‸‸‸‸‸‸‸‸‸‸‸‸

DAY 17

EARTHQUAKE

THE LONG CHAINS OF MOUNTAINS that form our Rocky Mountain and Sierra Madre ranges run down the main body of Mexico until they are near present-day Mexico City. There the mountains break their parallel lines and seem to bunch together in what is sometimes called the Aztec Knot. This geographic confluence creates an area of strong earthquakes.

The Aztecs saw the earthquake as one of their gods. It also formed one of the major time epochs of their calendar—which ended in a catastrophic earthquake, after which men of artistry and sensitivity emerged. The reminder of that major quake inspired the Aztecs to cultivate the sensitivity of the human prototypes that emerged after that epoch. The foods of this day are foods grown from the earth and give the power of this god.

Several vegetable dishes are the main meal of this day. The Nahua Squash is a typical Aztec recipe, and it was included since zucchini are available all year round in most places.

Symbol	*Food*	*Power*
EARTHQUAKE	VEGETABLES	SENSITIVITY

Principal Meal
  Chive Broth, p. 131
  Nahua Squash, p. 149
  Sweet Tamale Pie, p. 146
  Savory Frijoles Refritos, p. 141
  Nuts

Morning
  Morning Rain, p. 163
  Fruit: melon
  Sun Coins with honey, p. 170

Midmorning
   Juice
   Rolls
   Handful (⅓ cup) pumpkin seeds

Evening
   Vegetable Plate, p. 164
   Hot rolls

EARTHQUAKE—VEGETABLES

HEALTHY INGREDIENTS AND COMBINATIONS

The tomato and the sweet potatoes in the main meal are some of the vitamin A-rich vegetables that the American Cancer Society recommends as a nutrition aid against cancer. The combination of the vegetables, the corn maza in the tamale, and the pinto beans provides complete protein. The beans also provide carbohydrates and iron, magnesium, and zinc; they also enhance the protein in the nuts.

The tortillas (Sun Coins) provide carbohydrates and B vitamins and fiber. The nuts provide unsaturated fats and vitamin E.

The vegetable plate served at the end of the day provides vitamins A and C, plus carbohydrates and fiber.

Day 18

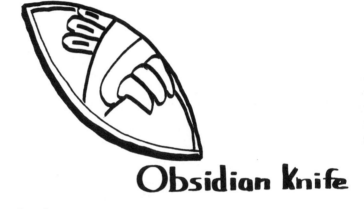

Obsidian Knife

Black knife of sorrow,
Black knife of regret,
Cut away from me my error,
Leave me renewed and changed.

Renewal......Power of Juice
                              Fast

DAY 18

OBSIDIAN KNIFE

FOR THE AZTECS, this was a special day dedicated to religious rites. No regular work was done and no market was held. It was a day to bring offerings and sacrifices to the temples. And as part of the religious focus of the day, no food was eaten, although juices of all kinds were taken.

In our culture and heritage, we do not commonly fast. People unaccustomed to doing so find the first day a difficult one in which they constantly think about how much they miss their regular foods. The Aztecs viewed the fast not from the perspective of what they were missing but of what they were gaining, since they felt that by this small act of self-denial they would gain the favor of their gods. After experiencing a fast day like this one several times, most people report that they feel more energetic than usual, and much more appreciative of the foods they take all the other days.

If you are not comfortable with this concept, then do not do this day as suggested. Eat moderately, using the menu from a day like Reed/Cane, for instance, with fish as the main meal, or a day like Wind, with vegetable tamales as the main meal. If for any reason you wonder if fasting is right for you, consult your physician before beginning any kind of fast. Anyone with diabetes or any condition that requires regular medication should definitely fast only with the approval of a physician.

Symbol	Food	Power
OBSIDIAN	JUICE	RENEWAL
KNIFE	CLEANSING	
(Holiday)	FAST	

Juices of various kinds are taken throughout the day, depending upon what fruits or juices are available and in season. Also drink generous amounts of water.

OBSIDIAN KNIFE—JUICE

The juices taken throughout the day provide vitamin C, which is associated with internal cleansing and healing. Also, water is to be taken along with the juices, at least 8 oz. every three hours.

Day 19

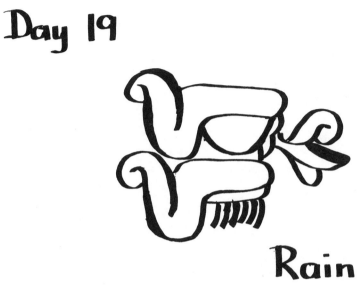

Rain

Silver shafts of falling rain
   Penetrate Mother Earth
To open seeds and sprout sweet fruit
   In the season of life.

Fertility . . . . . Power of Fruits

DAY 19

RAIN

SUMMER RAINS were absolutely vital to the crops. Tlaloc (TLAH-lock) was the god of rain, and his favors were diligently and carefully sought. The Aztecs believed that when he was angered there was no rain, and the resulting famine was his punishment. When properly honored, Tlaloc gave rain and gifts of fruit.

Many of the Aztecs' favorite fruits like mangoes, papayas, and guavas grew spontaneously in various parts of their empire. This day was a day in which fruits were eaten as the main meal, and fertility was the power gained.

The fruits in the Fruit Soup dish for today are more traditional to our climate, but still keep the spirit of the day. Rolls, which are not totally traditional Aztec fare, are such a pleasant accompaniment to this meal that I included them as part of the principal meal.

Symbol	*Food*	*Power*
RAIN	FRUITS	FERTILITY

Principal Meal
Fruit Soup, p. 136
Hot whole-wheat rolls served with honey

Morning
Morning Rain, p. 163
Fruit, mild, tropical: banana and papaya
Warm tortillas topped with honey

Midmorning
Juice
Honey Rolls, p. 164
Peanuts, raisins, sunflower seeds, shredded coconut, mixed (½ cup)

Evening
Fruit Compote, p. 170
Tortillas, warmed and served with honey

RAIN—FRUITS

HEALTHY INGREDIENTS AND COMBINATIONS

Fruit is the main food of this day, so at every meal there is a bountiful supply of vitamins C and A. Fruits such as bananas and papayas also provide potassium.

The fruits and rolls and tortillas provide carbohydrates and fiber along with B vitamins.

The fructose in the fruits provides a great deal of carbohydrates. The Aztecs felt that this day, along with the fruit day of Monkey, were "energizing" days, in response to the high amount of fructose.

Day 20

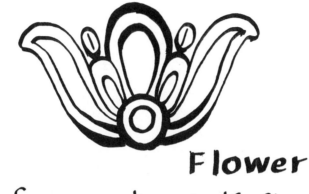

Flower

As fragrance lives in the flower
   And yields fruit,
So hope lives in my heart
   And yields peace.

Contentment..... Power of this
                     Feast

DAY 20

FLOWER

FLOWER IS A FEAST DAY. Flowers were extensively cultivated by the Aztecs. Netzahualcoyotl (Nets-ah-wall-COH-yottl), the poet-king of Texcoco who ruled from the 1430s to 1472, was a man of great architectural and engineering talents. He planned extensive aqueducts to bring fresh water to the region, and his botanical gardens were extensive and beautiful. Subsequent rulers kept this tradition of designating moneys from the state treasury for gardens. Flowers were appropriate religious offerings, and individual and commercial gardens were a part of Aztec tradition.

Often a wild pig (javalina) was served on a community feast day like Flower. The pig was roasted in a pit lined with very hot stones on the bottom and up the sides. The pig was cleaned and carefully wrapped in banana leaves, lowered into the pit and covered with more leaves, then covered with clean sand. It cooked from very early morning until afternoon. When dug out and unwrapped it was the scrumptious center of the feast.

The roast pork recipe given for this day is the most authentic food. Pork may not appeal to everyone, so turkey could be used again, even though it would be the third time in one month of the calendar.

Symbol	*Food*	*Power*
FLOWER	ROAST PORK or TURKEY (feast)	CONTENTMENT

Principal Meal
   Vegetable Soup, p. 132

   Javali, p. 160

                                    or

   Slow Roast Turkey, p. 157

   Sweet Little Tamales, p. 156
   Aztec Beans, p. 142
   Nopal Fritters, p. 168

Morning
>   Morning Rain, p. 163
>   Honey Rolls, p. 164
>   Fruits: coconut, banana

Midmorning
>   Tropical juices: papaya, guava, pineapple
>   Peanut brittle

Evening
>   Nahua Squash, p. 149
>   Pyramids, p. 144

FLOWER—PORK OR TURKEY

HEALTHY INGREDIENTS AND COMBINATIONS

The main meal of today's feast day begins with vegetable broth, which has vitamin A from the carrots.

The pork provides much animal (complete) protein and iron, thiamin, niacin, and vitamin B_6.

The Sweet Tamales yield B vitamins, carbohydrates, and calcium. In combination with the beans they provide additional complete protein, along with vitamin A and carbohydrate.

The morning fruits and midmorning tropical juices are a good supply of vitamin C. The accompanying rolls and honey provide additional B vitamins and a good supply of carbohydrates.

Recipes

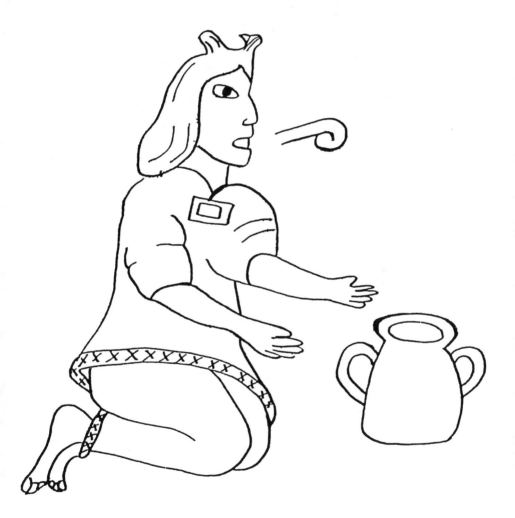

7
Recipes

It has been an engrossing challenge to present the recipes that accompany the Aztec Foods in as practical a way as possible. Regardless of how delicious and healthy any group of foods is, few will have their benefits if they are very difficult to prepare.

With that in mind, I have adapted and made substitutions that seemed to make sense given our facilities and products. In Aztec times foods were marketed directly with no freezing or canning, but I work outside my home, and have many of the same time limitations as most people I know. Therefore I have used many convenience products and suggest them in the recipes. I also take advantage of such appliances as a microwave, and suggest them in food preparation where it makes sense. As with any other foods, dishes made fresh at home are definitely more tasty. For example, if you have the time to prepare your own tortillas or fresh chilies, the wonderful fresh flavors will certainly enhance your meal, but you can gain most of the same flavor and nutrition by buying packaged tortillas and canned chilies.

My own family benefits most when our time and schedules allow us all to be home for the major midday meal. I have found several ways to change and adapt that basic feature of Aztec foods, and know that the options are limited only by the creativity of the individual. Use your creativity in making time variations and recipe variations to suit your taste.

After all, that is what the Aztecs (or any other group of people, for that matter) did. While any given ethnic foods have certain characteristic flavors or ingredients, some people within that group have more of a genuine talent for cooking than others. They are the ones who devise new recipes. If the recipes or preparation methods are good, they soon get copied and circulated.

If you decide to make your own variations, don't feel limited, remembering that the Aztec empire included a wide variety of climates and natural resources. Depending on location, many more things were actually eaten than are represented by the recipes suggested here, such as turtle and certain kinds of lizards and different fruits of certain cactuses. These items would certainly be authentic, but not practical or readily available.

Nine recipes use cream cheese, which I found to be useful in texture and mild enough in taste to provide the balance for the other ingredients. The amount of the cheese in any individual portion is not large enough to be a concern in terms of either calories or cholesterol, especially given the low-fat nature of all the foods in general. A mild-flavored nut butter such as almond butter is an interesting substitute if you want to keep a lactose-free diet. If you try it, whip the butter with an equal amount of a light margarine, such as corn or safflower, and use one tablespoon per ounce of cream cheese in a recipe.

In all the recipes, if you keep within the character of each day, you will probably find certain substitutions that please your palate and make the Aztec foods a real boost to your health, well-being, and sense of adventure.

All recipes serve four unless otherwise stated.

Soups

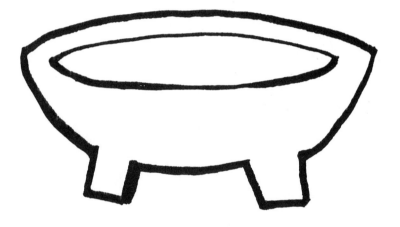

"AS EASY AS DUCK SOUP" *is an old saying that highlights the fact that soups are generally easy to prepare. Because the Aztecs made them light introductions to the meal, they are more broth-type then cream or hearty soups. That is why the preparation portion of these soup recipes is generally short, since the basic procedure is to gently simmer several ingredients to blend their tastes.*

CLEAR ONION/VEGETABLE (CHIVES) BROTH

4 cups water
1 medium tomato, cut into 1 inch-cubes
½ medium onion or 1 bunch chives or 8–10
    scallions, cut small
2 carrots, cut into 1-inch pieces
2–3 celery stalks, cut into 1-inch pieces
¼ tsp rosemary
¾ tsp salt (or to taste)

Add vegetables to water in medium-sized pan. Cook at a very low simmer for 1 to 1½ hours. Ladle into serving dishes.

THIS RECIPE *is a classic Mexican one, but substitutions can be made easily. The amount of any one ingredient is not large, and the soup may depend more on what is in your refrigerator than what is included in the recipe given here.*

VEGETABLE SOUP

3 cups water
Small bunch of scallions or chives
2 carrots, cut thin
3 tomatoes, diced
1 medium jicama, diced (substitute: 1 medium potato)
8–10 green beans, cut small
2–3 stalks celery, chopped fine
1 tsp parsley
½ tsp salt

Combine ingredients in medium pot that has a snug-fitting lid. Barely simmer over low heat for 1½ to 2 hours.

THIS IS A VERY MILD BROTH with a delicate flavor. The Aztecs would have served this in a bowl and then sipped it rather than eating it with a spoon, making the aroma part of the enjoyment. A soup mug preserves that tradition.

PARSLEY BROTH

4 cups water
1 medium onion, halved
2 cloves garlic, halved
3–4 peppercorns
½ bay leaf
¼ tsp marjoram
1 carrot, cut in 3 or 4 pieces
8 sprigs parsley
1 tomato, quartered
½ tsp salt

Combine all ingredients in a 3- to 4-quart pot. Simmer for 1½ hours. Serve the broth only.

THIS HEARTY SOUP is ready to serve in less than half an hour.

CORN SOUP

1 *medium onion*
½ *tsp chili powder*
3 *cups broth, chicken or vegetable*
2 *cups puréed, cooked sweet corn or 1 can cream-style*
corn
1 *tsp salt*
2 *tbs light oil (safflower, corn, or canola)*

Sauté the onion in the oil in a 3- to 4-quart pot. After 5 minutes, add the chili powder and continue to sauté over low heat for an additional 5 minutes.

Add the broth, corn, and salt. Simmer over very low heat for 10 to 15 minutes. (Don't let it boil or the corn will scorch on the bottom of the pan.)

THIS IS A RICH SOUP, *and the herbs and spices are very important to the overall flavor. It is important to blend the cream cheese with the squash so that the cheese is not lumpy. I usually use a blender, but have done this with a potato masher as well.*

BUTTERNUT SOUP WITH HERBS

6 *scallions*
2 *tsp* *fresh, peeled, grated ginger*
1 *tbs* *light oil (corn or safflower)*
3 *cups* *vegetable broth*
2 *cups* *puréed squash (butternut, acorn, or other*
sweet-meat squash; fresh, frozen, or canned)
4 *oz.* *cream cheese*
½ *tsp* *salt*
¼ *tsp* *nutmeg*
¼ *tsp* *rosemary*
¼ *tsp* *basil*
½ *tsp* *parsley*
1 *lime (a small squeeze for each serving)*

Sauté scallions and ginger in the tablespoon of oil. Add the broth and let it steep while you purée the squash with the cream cheese. Add to the broth. Add the remaining ingredients. Heat slowly until barely simmering. Just before serving, splash each individual serving with a small squeeze of lime juice.

THIS IS LIKE a very light fruit stew. The fruits have a small amount of natural thickening, and most mixtures cook to a deep gold color. Packages of dried fruit are usually in the same section of the grocery store as items like raisins.

FRUIT SOUP

1 lb. dried fruit mixture, diced (mixtures usually
            contain prunes, apples, apricots peaches,
            and pears)
4–5 cups water
3 tbs honey
½ tsp salt

Very gently simmer ingredients for approximately 1 hour in a covered 3-quart pot with a snug lid. Stir occasionally.

A garnish of ½ teaspoon crumbled dried mint leaves can be added on each serving.

THERE ARE AS MANY RECIPES *for tortilla soup as there are regions in Mexico. I like this one because it is easy to prepare. Fresh or frozen stock, if you have time to simmer some, makes this extra tasty (see p. 157).*

TORTILLA SOUP

        1 *clove garlic, minced*
        1 *large sweet green pepper, diced*
        2 *large tomatoes, diced*
    ¼ cup *light oil (corn or safflower)*
        4 *tortillas cut into 1-by-2-inch strips*
   3 cups *turkey or chicken stock or 1 can condensed*
            consommé plus 10 oz. water
    ½ cup *fresh mixed herbs: cilantro (coriander), chives,*
            basil, parsley
  1½ tsp *salt*
    3 tbs *lemon or lime juice*

Lightly sauté tortilla strips in oil. Add the garlic, green pepper, and tomatoes and salt. Cook for 5 minutes, stirring occasionally. Add stock and herbs and simmer gently for 20 minutes. Add lemon or lime juice and serve.

Main Dishes

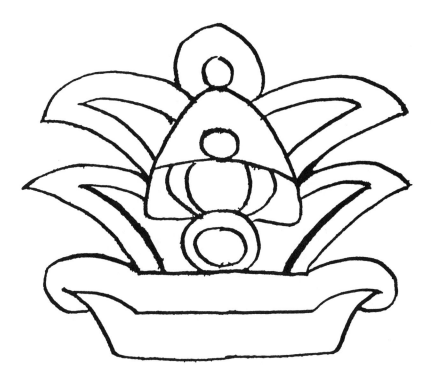

HUACHINANGO (Red Snapper)

3 medium tomatoes, diced
1 medium onion, chopped
3 tbs honey
½ cup mild chilies, diced
1 tsp salt
2 lb. red snapper

In a large skillet combine tomatoes, onion, honey, chilies, and salt. Cook over medium-low heat for 15 minutes, stirring frequently. Reduce heat to very low and add fish filets. Cover. Cook, turning once, approximately 20 minutes or until the fish flakes easily with a fork.

I AM ALWAYS DISCONCERTED to see "refried beans" as the common translation of Frijoles Refritos. In Spanish the prefix RE- not only means "again," it also means "very." In this case it means very or thoroughly, not "fried again."

SAVORY FRIJOLES REFRITOS

3 cups cooked pinto beans (recipe, p. 142) or use
canned refried beans
½ cup broth
¼ cup salsa (see recipe, p. 169, or use commercial
product, mild to hot to taste)
½ cup cream cheese

Combine broth and salsa in large skillet. Cook over low heat for 5 to 10 minutes. Add beans and mash thoroughly while continuing to cook over low heat. Add cream cheese. Cook 10 minutes, stirring frequently.

THIS RECIPE does not require a great deal of tender care. When I am in a hurry, I put everything in the pot part of the crock pot the night before and put it in the refrigerator. The next morning I just put the pot back in the cooker, set it to the lowest setting, and have the main meal ready later in the day.

PAINTED SQUASH STEW

4 cups water
1 small onion, diced
2 carrots cut into thin slices
1 sweet bell pepper, cut lengthwise and diced
3 stalks celery, cut thin
1 cucumber, diced
1 yellow squash, diced very small
1 cup cooked pinto beans
1½ tsp salt
Juice of ½ lemon (2 tbs)
½ tsp thyme

Add all ingredients in a pot with a tight-fitting lid (a crock pot is ideal). Simmer on very low setting for 2 or 2½ hours

---

AZTEC BEANS WITH MILD CHILIES

1 cup dried pinto or Anasazi beans
1 clove garlic
1 small onion
1 tsp salt
1 small (4 oz.) can mild chilies
1 cup crushed pineapple

Soak beans in water overnight. Rinse thoroughly, put them in a pot that has a snug lid, and add water to cover. Add garlic, onion, and salt. Cover and simmer until tender, 2 hours or more. Add chilies and pineapple and simmer 15 minutes more.

COOKING TIME CAN BE LENGTHENED *on this dish if the cooking temperature is low. It not only does well as a stovetop recipe or a crockpot recipe, it can also be cooked in the oven. The dish does well at 275 to 300 degrees for 5 to 6 hours.*

OLLA LAMB

2 or 3 *meaty lamb shanks*
3 *medium jicamas* or 4 *medium potatoes*
10 *scallions, including at least half green portion*
 of stalks, sliced thin
2 *cloves garlic, minced*
2 tbs *light cooking oil (corn, safflower, or canola)*
4 *carrots, cut small*
4–5 *stalks celery, sliced thin*
1 *sweet green pepper, cut lengthwise and diced*
2 *medium tomatoes, diced*
2 tsp *salt*

In a heavy stew pot, sauté scallions and garlic in oil for 10 minutes. Add lamb shanks and enough water to cover. Peel jicamas or potatoes and cut into bite-sized cubes and add to mixture. Add remaining ingredients and barely simmer for 2 to 3 hours. The resulting stew will be light rather than thick.

YOU CAN FIND MASA HARINA in the flour section in most super-markets. When you read the ingredients, you will see that it is made of corn that has been treated with lime water and specially milled. When you work with it, you will see that it is different than corn meal, which is more coarse, because it is indeed a flour, although it is a little grainy. It does not stick together or make a smooth dough the way wheat flour does because it lacks the gluten of wheat.

When you are making the crust for this dish, the consistency of the dough is quite variable, depending on the thickness of the creamed corn and the humidity. You can add extra masa if you think it is too runny, but the trick is not to add too much or the dough will behave like loose crumbs and not hold together. This kind of dough is not like flour piecrust, which is somewhat elastic and relatively dry. This dough is more moist, which is why you can just pat it into a crust.

This dish is called Pyramids because the mounded ingredients in the center resemble the low, four- to five-step pyramids that line the main thoroughfare of Teotihuacan.

PYRAMIDS

1½ cups masa harina (corn flour)
½ cup puréed sweet corn or canned cream-style
corn
4 oz. cream cheese
½ cup salsa, mild or hot to taste
2 tomatoes, sliced thin
2 sweet green peppers, cut small

Preheat oven to 350 degrees.

Mix the masa with ¾ cup of water and ½ cup of puréed or creamed corn to form a workable dough. Divide the dough into four portions. Pat each into a round crust on a piece of foil about 8 inches square. Fold the foil around the edges so the dough forms a raised edge. The foil will be thicker where the corners are rolled up, but that does not affect the dough.

Work the salsa into the cream cheese so the cheese is soft and easy to spread. Spread the cheese mixture into the dough circle. Add a thin layer of green pepper and two or three slices of tomato. Bake at 350 degrees for 20 minutes.

VEGETABLE TAMALE PIE

CRUST
>1¼ cups masa harina
>½ cup creamed corn
>⅓ to ½ cup water, enough to make a soft, pliable
>dough

FILLING
>3 medium-size zucchini
>⅓ cup tomato sauce
>1 cup broccoli flowerets
>2 eggs, separated
>8 oz. cream cheese
>1 tsp salt
>2 tbs chopped chives
>⅛ tsp pepper
>¼ tsp cream of tartar

Preheat oven to 400 degrees.

For the crust, combine ingredients and pat into an 8- or 9-inch pie plate. See note about making crusts with masa (p. 144). Expect to pat it into the pie plate since it does not form a cohesive sheet the way regular flour piecrust does.

For the filling, wash and slice zucchini and sauté in the tomato sauce for 15 minutes. In a blender, blend the cream cheese with enough water to give it the consistency of thick cream. Add broccoli and blend for 2 or 3 seconds.

In a bowl, beat the egg yolks, then add the cream cheese–broccoli mixture, salt, chives, and pepper.

In a separate bowl, beat the egg whites with the cream of tartar until stiff but not dry. Fold into the cream-cheese mixture. Place half the zucchini on the piecrust. Spoon over half of the cream-cheese mixture. Place remaining zucchini on top and cover with the remaining mixture. Bake at 400 degrees for 10 minutes; reduce setting to 325 degrees and continue baking for 45 to 50 minutes.

THIS IS ANOTHER RECIPE in which there is a masa crust (see note on page 144). When done, this dish will resemble a very moist pumpkin pie in texture and will be a rich, deep orange.

As for the size of cooking utensil—the Aztecs used pottery baking dishes and shells from large marine animals, such as abalone, all of which varied in size. Either size will do—in the recipes that suggest an 8-by-10-inch dish, it was probably because my oven sets vary also, and I found the slightly smaller size to be ideal.

SWEET TAMALE PIE

CRUST

    1¼ cups masa harina
    ½ cup creamed corn
    ⅓ to ½ cup water, enough to make a soft, pliable dough

FILLING

    5 medium sweet potatoes.
    2 medium ripe bananas or 1 large
    1½ tbs melted margarine
    ½ tsp salt
    1 egg, beaten

Preheat oven to 350 degrees.

Combine ingredients for crust and pat into a 9- or 10-inch pie plate or shallow 8-by-11-inch baking dish.

Cook sweet potatoes in boiling water for 30 minutes. Peel and mash until there are only a few small lumps left. Mash in the remaining ingredients and spoon into crust. Bake at 350 degrees for 20 to 25 minutes.

FRUIT SKEWERS

3 *bananas*
1 *fresh pineapple*
2 *oranges*
2 *apples*
1 *mango*
1 *papaya*
  (canned peach halves can be substituted for the
  papaya and mango)

Slice bananas into thick pieces. Cube or section other fruit to a similar size. Coat with a mixture of ⅓ cup honey and ¼ cup orange juice. Place on skewers and broil for 5 to 7 mins.

THIS IS ONE of Mexico's most famous dishes. The chocolate does not add a sweet flavor. In this dish, combined with the flavor of the coriander and cinnamon, it has an interesting, smoky taste.

TURKEY MOLE

4 turkey thighs
1 sweet bell pepper, diced
1 can diced chili peppers
2 tbs sesame seeds, toasted
¼ cup peanuts, roasted
2 tomatoes, diced
½ tsp salt
¼ tsp coriander
½ tsp cinnamon
2 tbs masa harina
½ ounce unsweetened chocolate, grated

Preheat oven to 325 degrees.

Place the turkey thighs in a pot with just enough water to cover them and gently simmer for 1 hour. Remove from stock and set aside in a covered baking dish.

To stock add peppers, seeds and nuts, tomatoes and seasonings. Simmer for 15 minutes, shaking in masa harina to thicken. Pour sauce over turkey. Bake in a covered baking dish at 325 degrees for 2 hours.

Just before serving, pour or spoon off most of the sauce into a small saucepan over low heat. Add the chocolate to the heated sauce, stir quickly, pour evenly over the meat, and serve.

THIS IS A LIGHT, *refreshing way to prepare this wonderful vegetable that is so abundant in the summer. You can also substitute yellow crookneck squash or spaghetti squash, cutting the lengthwise strands into 2- to 3-inch pieces.*

A nice variation is to substitute 1 small jicama (about 4 inches across) for the onion and add 2 teaspoons crushed fresh or dried mint.

NAHUA SQUASH

2 small tomatoes, diced
1 small onion, diced
2 medium zucchini, diced
¼ cup crushed pineapple
½ tsp salt
½ tsp basil

Sauté all ingredients together over medium-low heat for 10 minutes, then cover and continue to barely simmer over very low heat for 20 minutes.

CAZUELA OF CASSAVA OR SWEET POTATO

1 small onion, diced
1 clove of garlic, minced
2 tbs cooking oil
2 tbs honey
3 medium sweet potatoes, peeled and cubed
2 15-oz. cans creamed corn
¼ cup (approximately) masa harina
¼ tsp marjoram
¼ tsp coriander
½ tsp salt

Sauté onion and garlic in oil for 10 minutes. Add potatoes and enough water to barely cover, and cook covered until potatoes are tender. Add the honey, creamed corn, and spices. Continue cooking over low heat for 15 minutes. Add masa harina 1 tablespoon at a time to bring to desired consistency, stirring constantly, then serve.

THIS IS A VERY POPULAR DISH in Mexico today, and goes by a number of names, the best-known being Huevos Rancheros. In some locales it is just as popular for breakfast as any other time.

Cooking the beans with the honey gives them an unexpected sweet flavor, which combines well with the eggs and salsa.

FEATHERED SERPENT BEANS

1 cup   dried pinto or Anasazi beans
1   medium onion, diced
1 tsp   salt (or to taste)
4   tomatoes, diced
½ to 1 tsp   chili powder, to taste
6 tbs   honey
12–15   cilantro (coriander) leaves

1 or 2   eggs per person
Mild salsa (p. 169, or commercial product)

Soak beans overnight in enough water to have 4 to 5 inches of water above the top of the beans. Rinse thoroughly.

Place in a 4-quart pot with water to cover well. Add the other ingredients except the eggs and salsa; cook over low heat until the beans are very tender, 2 to 3 hours. Mash very lightly. Serve topped with one or two eggs over easy, garnished liberally with a mild salsa.

ARM YOURSELF WITH PATIENCE *as you scoop the squash out of its shell. I try to use a spoon that has a thin rim rather than a paring knife. I have better luck leaving the skin intact that way, which is worth the effort as this is such a festive dish with the colorful tomatoes and peppers.*

SQUASH BOATS

2 *large yellow or zuccini squash*
2 *small tomatoes, diced*
1 *sweet bell pepper, diced small*
3 *stalks celery, diced very small*
½ tsp *salt*
*Small (4-oz.) can diced chilies or ½ cup fresh chilies**
4 oz. *cream cheese*

Preheat oven to 350 degrees.

Cut squash in half lengthwise. Scoop out seeds and discard. Scoop out most of the meat, being careful not to mar the skin. Dice meat and place in a 10- to 12-inch skillet. Add tomatoes, peppers, celery, and chilies. Sauté in their own juices over low heat until squash is tender.

Mix in cream cheese and stir frequently until the cheese is blended through.

Return this mixture to squash shells, then bake at 350 degrees for 20 to 30 minutes.

* This makes a relatively spicy dish. You can vary this by decreasing the amount or spiciness of the chilies.

DEEP DISH CORN

¼ cup stock or water
5–6 scallions, cut fine
1 sweet green pepper, diced fine
2½ cups corn cut from very tender ears or 1 can
(17 oz.) cream-style corn
⅓ cup corn meal
¼ tsp salt
¼ tsp sage
¼ tsp basil
2 eggs, beaten well

Preheat oven to 375 degrees.

In a 12-inch skillet, gently simmer onion and pepper in the stock or water until tender. Remove from heat, and then add the remaining ingredients, making sure the eggs are added last, when mixture is cooler. Pour into a greased 4-quart casserole or baking dish. Bake at 375 degrees for approximately 40 minutes.

BITTERSWEETS

½ cup chicken stock or water
6–8 scallions, cut fine
1 sweet green pepper, cut fine
1 lb. chicken livers, cut in small pieces
½ tsp salt
2 tbs honey
1½ cups crushed pineapple

In a 12-inch skillet, sauté scallions and green pepper in water or stock over a low flame. Add livers, salt, and honey. Cook until tender. Add pineapple and cook 5 minutes longer.

Serve over Corn Bread (p. 165) sliced lengthwise.

TAMALE CASSEROLE

  1 *lb.* *ground meat*
  ½ *tsp salt*
  ¼ *tsp thyme*
  1 *tsp cumin*
     10 *ears fresh corn or 2 cans (15 oz. each) cream-
        style corn*
  1 *pkg. corn husks, if needed (usually available in the
        specialty section at the supermarket)*
  1 *cup cornmeal*
  1 *can diced green chilies*

Preheat oven to 350 degrees.

Brown ground meat with salt, thyme, and cumin and set aside. Shuck corn and save husks. Cut kernels from cobs and grind in blender. Put puréed corn or canned creamed corn in a bowl and add enough corn meal to make a mixture that can be spread easily.

Place a layer of corn husks in a 4-quart casserole or an 8-by-10-inch baking dish, making sure that the husks extend up the sides. Spoon about half of corn purée over husks, then the ground meat. Spread the chilies over the meat, then add the other half of the corn purée. Cover with foil and bake at 350 degrees for about one hour.

To serve, scoop the casserole off the corn husks and onto your plate.

SPICY CHICKEN

1 *frying chicken (2½–3 lbs.), or 2½–3 lbs.*
rabbit meat
½ *cup corn meal*
¼ *cup amaranth or whole-wheat flour*
1–2 *tsp chili powder or to taste*
¼ *tsp garlic powder*
½ *tsp salt*
½ *tsp ground cumin*

Preheat oven to 400 degrees.

Run chicken pieces under water to freshen and moisten, then skin them (rabbit comes skinned). Combine corn meal, flour, and spices. Roll the meat in the corn-meal mixture. Place in a shallow 8-by-10-inch baking dish and bake at 400 degrees for about 45 minutes.

THIS DISH CAN BE TIME-CONSUMING to prepare, but it freezes very well. I often double the ingredients and serve it as a company meal. I fix it whenever convenient, then cover well and freeze. If I am putting it directly from freezer to oven, I cover the outside edges of the baking dish with foil, bringing the foil over the filling by 2 or 3 inches so that the tortillas don't get too crisp.

SOARING WINGS

¾ lb. *lean ground meat*
1 *small onion, diced fine*
¾ tsp *salt*
¼ tsp *garlic powder*
¼ tsp *cilantro (coriander)*
1 *large (29 oz.) can tomato sauce*
½ cup *mild salsa (p. 169)*
12 *tortillas*
8 oz. *cream cheese* or *3 sliced bananas*
½ cup *diced chilies (4-oz. can), mild or hot to taste*

Preheat oven to 350 degrees.

In a large frying pan, brown the meat with the onion, salt, garlic, and cilantro. Add the salsa and 1 cup of the tomato sauce. Simmer for 15 minutes over low heat.

Soften tortillas in microwave or in a moistened, closed paper sack in a 350-degree oven for 10 minutes.

Use six of the tortillas to line the bottom of a shallow 8-by-11-inch baking dish (the pan size is approximate), arranging them so the edges come up the sides of the baking dish. Cover with half of the meat mixture. Cut the cream cheese as thin as practical (or slice the bananas into thin slices). Add half of the cheese or bananas and half of the chiles, spreading them evenly over the meat mixture. Cover with the remaining tortillas, then add the rest of the meat mixture and the remaining cheese or bananas and chilies. Spread evenly. Spread the remainder of the tomato sauce over the top. Bake at 350 degrees for 30 to 45 minutes.

SWEET LITTLE TAMALES

1½ cup masa harina
1½ cup puréed sweet corn or 1 can cream-style corn
   4 oz. cream cheese or ½ cup mashed banana
  2 tsp salsa (p. 169), mild or hot
  2 tbs honey
  1 pkg. corn husks (optional)

Preheat oven to 350 degrees.

Mix the masa with ¾ cup of water and ½ cup of the creamed corn to form a workable dough. Pat into a thin crust in three overlapping broad corn husks or on a piece of aluminum foil about 12 inches wide. Pat dough into a thin crust in a 5-by-10-inch rectangle. Combine cheese, salsa, and honey and put as a filling in the dough. Cover with an equal rectangle of thin dough and cover with three or four overlapping husks and tie with a string or cover with the foil, sealing the edges. Bake at 350 degrees for 45 or 50 minutes.

SLOW ROAST TURKEY

1 *whole turkey, 10 to 12 lbs.*
2 *tsp salt*
1 *tsp sage*
1 *tsp thyme*
1 *tsp basil*
1 *tsp garlic powder*

Rinse inside cavity of the turkey, and rinse skin also, to freshen and moisturize. In a small bowl, mix salt and spices. Rub inside of cavity with this mixture and sprinkle liberally on the skin.

Place turkey inside a brown paper grocery sack, then place this sack inside a second sack with the open end of the first sack facing the bottom end of the second sack. Place in a shallow pan that has some sort of roasting rack.

Do not preheat the oven, since that activates the top heating element, which could burn the sacks.

Do not use a broiler.

Bake at 300 degrees, calculating 45 minutes per pound of turkey. To serve, just tear open and discard sacks and place turkey on a serving platter.

I use the carcass of the turkey and any leftover meat to make a stock or broth.

Break the carcass into convenient sections, put them in a medium or large pot and cover up to about three-quarters of the bones. Barely simmer for about an hour. Pour off the resulting stock through a clean, open-weave cloth or a very-fine-mesh metal strainer. Put into a freezable container and freeze until needed.

158 THE AZTEC WAY TO HEALTHY EATING

AS WITH MANY DISHES and snacks in Mexico, this dish is eaten with the fingers. Pick up the rolled-up tortilla, tuck the bottom end in so the sauce does not drip, and enjoy!

MAZATLES

1 lb. beef tenderloin tips or kebob squares, cut thin
½ medium onion, diced
1 clove garlic, minced
1 sweet green pepper, diced
3 stalks celery, diced
2 tbs cooking oil
½ cup broth
¼ cup dark molasses
½ tsp thyme
½ tsp dried cilantro (coriander)
½ tsp basil
½ tsp chili powder or to taste

1 dozen tortillas

Sauté meat, onion, garlic, pepper, and celery in the cooking oil until meat is browned. Then add the broth, molasses, and seasonings. Simmer for 15 to 20 minutes, stirring frequently. Soften tortillas (see p. 170). Place about 2 tablespoons of meat sauce in center of tortilla and roll loosely.

GOLDEN FISH

1½–2 lbs. *light fish such as perch, cod, or haddock*
½ tsp *salt*
1 tbs *light cooking oil (corn, safflower, or
    canola)*

SAUCE
¼ cup *margarine*
⅓ cup *honey*
¼ cup *lemon juice*
¼ tsp *thyme*

Sauté fish in cooking oil over very low heat. Sprinkle in salt as it begins to cook. In a saucepan, melt margarine over very low heat. Add honey, lemon juice, and thyme and continue to stir frequently for 5 minutes. Then pour over the fish and cook for 5 minutes more over low heat.

FOR THE MOST AUTHENTIC TASTE, scrub the potatoes and zucchini or summer squash thoroughly but do not peel. The jicama must be peeled, since the skin is tough and leathery. When testing the potatoes for doneness, use a table fork. When it goes into the potato easily, the dish is done. Do watch carefully, however, to make sure that what you have is a piece of potato and not the similar-looking jicama, because the jicama stays crisp even after cooking.

CALDO BUENO

½ lb. *lean ground beef*
1 *clove garlic, minced*
½ tsp *salt*
1 *large can (29 oz.) tomatoes*
3 *medium white or red potatoes, diced*
1 *medium jicama (4 to 5 inches across), diced*
3 *medium summer squash or zucchini, diced*
2 cups *sweet corn kernels*
1 tsp *oregano*
¼ cup *fresh parsley*

Brown meat, garlic, and salt in a heavy stew pot. Add remaining ingredients and enough water to cover. Simmer gently for about half an hour, until potatoes are done.

JAVALI

1 *pork tenderloin (4 to 5 lb.)*
1 tsp *salt*
¼ tsp *rosemary*
½ tsp *crushed coriander seed*
1 tbs *flour*

Preheat oven to 350 degrees.

Score the top of the roast with cuts about 1 inch apart and ½ inch deep. Mix seasonings and flour together and press into cuts. Make a foil tent and cover the top of the roast. Roast at 350 degrees, allowing 30 to 35 minutes per pound.

Side Steps

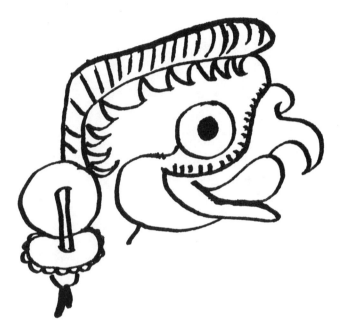

THE CUSTOM *of Morning Rain is an important part of the Aztec foods and will start your morning in a gentle and pleasant way.*

MORNING RAIN

Large glass
3 oz. any kind of fruit juice
9 oz. warm to slightly hot water

Stir

AZTEC MUFFINS

½ cup sourdough starter
3 oz. warm water
¼ cup cornmeal
1¼ cups amaranth or whole-wheat flour
pinch of salt

Mix together the sourdough starter and water. Add all but 1 tablespoon of the corn meal and the salt and mix well. Turn out onto a lightly floured surface and knead till smooth and elastic. Roll dough to a ⅜-inch thickness. Let rest a few minutes.

Us a 3-inch cutter and cut into muffins. Sprinkle a small cookie sheet with the remaining corn meal and put the muffins on it, then sprinkle additional corn meal on the tops. Cover with a clean cloth. Let rise about 45 minutes.

Bake on medium-hot griddle. (Spray with no-stick shortening for ease of baking and clean-up.) Turn every 5 minutes. Bake until lightly browned, about 30 minutes. Makes 7 to 8.

VEGETABLE PLATE

Both hot and cold vegetables can be served for this dish.

A typical cold vegetable plate would have three vegetables, often of different colors, sliced and laid on the plate in some alternating order or attractive design. An example would be slices of cucumber, jicama, and tomatoes.

A typical hot vegetable plate would have two or three steamed vegetables, such as carrots, broccoli, and pearl onions, sprinkled with lemon juice and tossed together.

HONEY ROLLS

2½ to 3 cups of amaranth or whole-wheat flour
1 cup sourdough starter
½ cup warm water
3 tbs honey
1 tsp salt

Combine 1 cup of the flour, the water, honey, and salt with the sourdough starter. Mix well with mixer, beating for 3 to 4 minutes.

Add enough of the remaining flour to make a spongy ball. Turn out on floured surface and knead well. Place in greased bowl and let rise for about 45 minutes, or until double. Form into balls, then pat into a circle about 4 inches in diameter. Place on ungreased baking sheet and bake at 400 degrees or till puffed, about 7 to 9 minutes. Cool on cloth-covered surface. Makes 12 to 15 rolls. Break puff and fill with honey when served.

CORN BREAD

½ cup corn meal
½ cup amaranth or whole-wheat flour
  2 eggs, beaten well
  ¼ cup water (or enough liquid to make a
      medium batter)
  3 tbs honey

Preheat oven to 400 degrees.

Mix ingredients together, then pour into a 9-inch-square greased baking pan. Bake at 400 degrees for 30 to 35 minutes. The bread will be thin and heavy.

Coat with honey while still warm.

I HAVE NOT FOUND a substitute for the cream cheese in this recipe that will yield the same texture.

AZTEC OMELETTE

  3 Aztec Muffins (substitute: English muffins)
  8 eggs
4 oz. cream cheese or 3 bananas, mashed
  1 small can diced chilies (mild)
½ tsp salt
  2 tomatoes, diced

Split muffins and place in a lightly greased, 8-by-11-inch shallow baking dish. Beat eggs lightly and add half of the cream cheese cut into very small pieces or the bananas. Spread the remaining half of the cheese or the bananas evenly on each of the muffins. Add chilies and salt to the egg mixture and pour this over the muffins. Garnish the top with the diced tomatoes.

Bake in a preheated oven at 350 degrees for 20 minutes.

SWEET ROLLED TORTILLAS

3 ounces cream cheese
¼ cup honey (or to taste)
6 tortillas

Thoroughly mix honey into cream cheese. Spread on tortillas and then roll them. Warm and serve. The microwave oven is ideal: Warm them on high for 20 seconds individually. To heat them all at once, arrange them so they are next to each other on a microwavable plate, set oven to 50 percent power, and warm for 1 minute 30 seconds, rotating at 45 seconds.

SWEET POCKETS

3 eggs, slightly beaten
2 cups cooked or canned pumpkin
½ cup honey
½ tsp salt
1 tsp cinnamon
¼ tsp nutmeg

Pie dough for 3 shells

In a large bowl, mix all of the ingredients except for the pie dough.

Roll out dough as though for pie. Cut into 4-inch circles. Place enough filling in the center of the circle to stuff it, approximately 2 tablespoons. Fold the circle in half and crimp the loose edges. Bake for 30 minutes at 350 degrees. These are done when they are a light golden brown.

TOMATO TOSTADA

3 *medium tomatoes, diced*
4 *scallions, cut fine*
3 *tbs honey*
¼ *tsp salt*
1 *tbs lime juice*
6 *warmed tortillas*

Slice tomatoes and scallions fine and heat in a heavy skillet over low heat for approximately 10 minutes. Add honey, salt, and lime juice and continue cooking an additional 5 minutes, stirring frequently. Serve over warmed tortillas (p. 170) or warmed commercial tostada shells.

LIKE MAZATLES (p. 158), this kind of dish can be served as a finger food. Hold the rolled tortilla carefully, folding up the bottom to keep the filling from dripping.

TURKEY TORTILLA ROLLS

1 *cup water, turkey stock, or drippings*
2 *tomatoes, diced small*
½ *tsp salt*
2 *tbs salsa, or to taste*
1–2 *tbs masa harina*
2 *cups cooked turkey meat, cut small*
1 *dozen tortillas*

In a heavy skillet combine water or broth, tomato, salt, and salsa. Cook over medium heat for 10 minutes. Add masa harina to thicken to the consistency of a thick sauce. Add turkey and heat thoroughly. Warm tortillas until they are soft (see p. 170), then place some turkey sauce in each tortilla and roll. Serve hot.

TOMATO, JICAMA, AND CHIVE MARINADE

2 medium tomatoes
1 medium jicama
1 small bunch chives or tender scallions
2 tbs lime juice
2 tbs honey

Dice tomatoes, jicama, and chives. Add lime juice, mix well, and let stand for at least an hour. Add the honey just before serving. Can be served chilled or at room temperature. It is more crisp when chilled, more authentic at room temperature.

NOPAL FRITTERS

2½ cups applesauce
2 tsp amaranth or whole wheat flour
¼ tsp salt
1 egg, separated

Beat egg yolk until creamy yellow. Add applesauce, flour, and salt. Whip the egg white until it will hold a stiff peak. Gently fold the egg white into the applesauce mixture.

Spoon batter in thin rounds on hot, greased griddle. Turn when bottom is golden brown, approximately 1½ to 2 minutes. Serve with honey.

MIXED VEGETABLES WITH TOMATO SALSA

1 16-oz. pkg. frozen mixed vegetables
1 medium tomato, sliced
1–2 tsp salsa, to taste (see p. 169)

Prepare vegetables according to package directions. In small saucepan, combine tomato and salsa and heat. Salsa should add only a mild flavor. Mix in with vegetables and serve.

THIS IS THE VERY BASIC BEGINNING of a salsa recipe. There are as many variations as cooks, since every person likes to add his or her own variations. Some like to make it sweeter by adding more tomatoes and some honey. Some like to add several other unique ingredients, such as half a shredded carrot or two colors of sweet peppers. There is a small green Mexican tomato called a tomatillo and some feel that is the proper tomato to use instead of the traditional red one from the store. Enjoy trying your own variations until you find the blend that suits you perfectly.

SALSA

8 tomatoes, diced
1–2 chili peppers to taste, seeds and membranes
   removed
1 large white onion, diced fine
2 tsp cilantro
⅓ cup vinegar
⅓ cup brown sugar
2 tsp salt

Put all ingredients into medium-size pot. Simmer over very low heat for 2 or 3 hours, until mixture is very thick. Adds spicy touch to any dish.

PALM TREAT TORTILLAS

2 bananas
½ cup shredded coconut
2 tbs honey
¼ tsp vanilla
5–6 corn tortillas

Mash bananas with coconut, honey, and vanilla. Spread on tortillas and roll tortillas. Warm individually for 15 seconds on high in a microwave oven.

FRUIT COMPOTE

Select your favorite fruits, especially those currently in season. Peel and cut as necessary to serve in bite-sized pieces and serve in small, individual containers. Just before serving, season very lightly with lime juice.

SUN COINS

Tortillas (corn tortillas)—Sun Coins—are the staple grain of the Aztec foods.

When purchased in the store, they are usually in a plastic wrapper. Check for freshness by seeing how easily you can bend them. If they are fresh, they bend easily.

They are neither tasty nor appealing when they are cold. There are several ways to warm them.

One is to put them them in a small plastic sandwich baggie, fold the top over, and put them in the microwave. Three tortillas take about 1 minute on high.

Another is to lay them one at a time on a hot griddle for 20 to 30 seconds until they are soft and hot.

With the current popularity of Southwestern decor and objects, it is increasingly easy to purchase a clay "tortilla warmer," which should have a close-fitting lid. Put in a conventional oven at 325 degrees for 15 to 20 minutes for a thin-walled warmer, 30 minutes for a thicker-walled warmer, and the tortillas will be soft and will stay warm.

You can warm up to a dozen this way, which is an advantage, since you keep the stack warm while you are fixing or eating them one at a time.

Recipe Index

V